Communication and Community Engagement in Disease Outbreaks

Erma Manoncourt • Rafael Obregon
Ketan Chitnis
Editors

Communication and Community Engagement in Disease Outbreaks

Dealing with Rights, Culture, Complexity, and Context

Springer

Editors
Erma Manoncourt
Management & Development Consulting, Inc
Las Vegas, NV, USA

Rafael Obregon
UNICEF, Asunción, Paraguay

Ketan Chitnis
UNICEF Mozambique
Maputo, Mozambique

Disclaimer: The contents of the book do not represent the views of UNICEF nor WHO, only of the authors.

ISBN 978-3-030-92295-5 ISBN 978-3-030-92296-2 (eBook)
https://doi.org/10.1007/978-3-030-92296-2

This Springer imprint is published by the registered company Springer Nature Switzerland AG
The registered company address is: Gewerbestrasse 11, 6330 Cham, Switzerland

"This book is exceptionally timely given the current COVID-19 pandemic and humanitarian consequences and will be of interest to professionals, students, and academics. There is not another book that covers this important topic so comprehensively and the editors and contributors bring substantial credibility having direct experience of disease outbreaks and being leading thinkers in the field. The book places communication and engagement at its heart, showing how a sensitivity to culture, context and human rights can strengthen risk communication. The summary of the lessons learned, conclusions, and recommendations are an especially valuable contribution to improve future disease outbreak responses."

—**Glenn Laverack**. Visiting Professor,
Department of Sociology and Social Research, University of Trento, Italy;
Member—WHO Technical Advisory Group on Behavioural Insights and Sciences for Health

"As a practitioner with experience in several public health emergencies, I find this book to be both useful and usable. It is useful because it gives synthesized insights emerging from multiple outbreaks in a range of complex contexts. The chapters are "usable" because they are both concise and pragmatic. They save time for practitioners who would otherwise need to read several streams of literature across multiple disciplines. The concrete lessons provided through the compelling mix of perspectives from academics and practitioners (and many "academic-practitioners") are a great resource for converting insights into action."

—**Karen Greiner**, Regional Advisor, Social and Behavior Change,
UNICEF West and Central Africa Regional Office, Dakar, Senegal

"The book makes a timely and important contribution to the understanding and application of one of the most important challenges that researchers and practitioners in health and development face at a global and local level in the face of pandemics such as COVID-19, and which has been largely absent in many of the communication responses in different countries: community engagement. Challenges posed by the diverse collection of chapters that document responses to various outbreaks transcend risk communication and community engagement (RCCE), and delve into the need for operational definitions, measures, and explanatory models of culture and health, beyond the use of culturally appropriate messages and culturally sensitive communication towards critical approaches that advocate for culture-centred and participatory frameworks in which the involvement and voice of affected communities and human rights serve as a basic foundation to frame communication processes."

—**Jair Vega Casanova**, Professor, Department of Social Communication,
Universidad del Norte Barranquilla, Colombia;
Participant in The Communication and Community Engagement Group,
Independent Panel for Pandemic Preparedness and Response—WHO

Preface

Five years after the Ebola outbreak in West Africa shocked the world, the COVID-19 pandemic, once again, brought to the forefront of the international agenda on health security and global preparedness and response against pandemics the central role that issues such as community engagement, risk communication, misinformation and disinformation, and trust play in the implementation of effective actions to control and respond to infectious disease outbreaks. The COVID-19 pandemic also underscored the centrality of other issues such as the tensions between individual and collective rights and public health decisions that require the implementation, amongst other measures, of restrictions to move and travel freely. More importantly, however, the COVID-19 pandemic also has shown that in the context of infectious disease outbreaks and pandemic response, these issues do not operate in isolation. Rather, they are often highly interconnected and thus increasingly pose tremendous challenges to decision makers, public health professionals and communities, families, and individuals across regions and countries.

Yet, these challenges are not entirely new. The 2014–2015 Ebola outbreak in West Africa made clear that greater and urgent attention to risk communication and community engagement (RCCE) was required, as well as more investments and sustained efforts towards building readily available capacity at global, national, and local levels. The years that followed the Ebola outbreak led to an intense period of policy discussions, research initiatives, academic papers and programmatic models, frameworks, and platforms that, arguably, should have better prepared the world for future outbreaks and pandemics such as COVID-19.

After 2014, based on the lessons learned from the Ebola outbreak, multiple initiatives were launched, many of which were subsequently supported by lessons learned from the Zika outbreak. Amongst the most noticeable on that list includes the Ebola Anthropology Network, which transitioned into the Social Science in Humanitarian Action Platform; the Risk Communication and Community Engagement Collective Service, co-led by several international agencies; the GloPID-R Social Science Working Group, which advocates for greater use of social sciences into pandemic response; the WHO COVID-19 Roadmap Social Sciences in Outbreak Response Working Group; and the WHO Technical Advisory Group on

Behavioural Insights and Sciences for Health, which provides advice to the WHO on the integration of behavioural perspectives into its work. While these initiatives approach pandemics and outbreaks from relatively different conceptual and theoretical angles, they all converge around the strengthening of risk communication and community engagement.

While these initiatives have made important headway, especially in terms of global coordination, bolder advocacy for inclusion of RCCE in global and regional response frameworks, and some efforts aimed at strengthening local capacities, it is also true that a lot more remains to be done, especially to ensure that RCCE is optimally integrated in national and local responses. Limited financial investments in RCCE capacity and coordination of the RCCE responses remain as critical challenges. Indeed, throughout the months-long, and potentially years-long, response to the COVID-19 pandemic, we continue to hear calls for greater emphasis on risk communication and community engagement, especially to properly engage local communities, introduce or change behaviours quickly, build public trust in the response, and address misinformation and disinformation. Why has this, it seems, become a repeated mantra throughout and after pandemics or in the context of public health emergencies of international concern (PHEIC)? What is missing from global and country-level preparedness and pandemic response efforts to ensure that the world and countries alike are in a better position to address the social and behavioural aspects of the increasing number of public health emergencies more quickly, predictably, and effectively? While it would be pretentious to think that we can provide a definitive answer, we put forward a series of arguments that we believe may be missing from current efforts in pandemic preparedness and response, or that at least must be considered more deliberately.

In simple terms, we put forward three arguments. The first argument focuses on the need to seriously look at pandemic preparedness and response more holistically, through approaches that bring together multiple dimensions of human behaviour that are often seen as ancillary to the golden standards of evidence-based interventions in disease outbreak response. Building on Chap. 1, which provides a conceptual framework that draws on concepts such as risk communication and community engagement, culture, human rights, complexity, trust, and information and disinformation, this book focuses primarily on the human cultural and public dimensions of disease outbreak preparedness and response. In particular, the case studies featured in this book explore those concepts through different responses ranging from global to regional to national outbreaks.

The second argument focuses on the need to consider issues such as risk communication and community engagement, misinformation and disinformation, and trust-building, amongst others, equally across all types of responses to disease outbreaks and pandemics—small- and medium-scale response to disease outbreaks may provide the best opportunities to strengthen capacities, build systems, and develop relationships with communities that may become critical in large-scale responses, including pandemics. Thus, several case studies featured in this book look at these concepts through the lens of disease outbreaks that have not reached the prominence of outbreaks such as Ebola, Zika, and COVID-19. These include examples such as cholera and polio. We know very well that engaging communities, building trust, and changing behaviours or increasing adherence to preventive behaviours become very challenging during a pandemic or an outbreak.

The third argument focuses on the need to, once and for all, shift the focus of global and national-level initiatives towards preparedness instead of what remains as a primary emphasis on response. The cost of responding to the Ebola, Zika, and COVID-19 outbreaks/pandemic together may be impossible to calculate but, arguably, the investments needed to have prepared systems and communities for such complex events may have cost just a fraction of it. Such an effort requires an in-depth review of the current global architecture in risk communication and community engagement, a greater emphasis on the integration of the concepts included in the framework we put forward into public health systems, and greater investments and strategic actions to operationalize the implementation of that framework, especially at national and local levels.

This book is organized into three parts. Part I—Conceptual Framework (Chaps. 1–3) provides the conceptual underpinnings. Chapter 1 introduces critical concepts that lead to the development of a conceptual framework that serves as a reference for the case studies included in the book. Chapter 2 provides a critical review of the global architecture in infectious disease outbreak and pandemic response with a focus on the need to further integrate key concepts outlined in Chap. 1 in global and country-level capacity strengthening efforts. Lastly, Chap. 3 provides a rich overview of what is perhaps the central element to strengthening country-level preparedness and response—community engagement—including a focus towards a common nomenclature and understanding of what community engagement means in pandemic and disease outbreak response.

Part II—Case Studies: Learning from Practice (Chaps. 4–9) features a collection of case studies that draw on real and practical experiences in disease outbreak and pandemic preparedness and response—large and small scale. Chapter 4 discusses the behavioural interventions needed to prepare for and respond to polio outbreaks by highlighting successful initiatives and comparing them to key challenges faced, depending on the region and country. In Chap. 5, the authors discuss the role of Risk Communication and Community Engagement interventions in the Ebola preparedness and response in eastern and southern Africa. Emphasis is placed on examining the influence of context, culture, trust, complexity, and rights dimensions on social and behaviour during the Ebola outbreak. As a complement, Chap. 6 expands the reflection by analysing the Ebola outbreak response in West Africa, specifically Sierra Leone, and by examining, in-depth, how leveraging community assets made a difference in the overall response. Chapter 7 addresses the Zika outbreak in the Americas and centres on the US Government's international response in Latin America and the Caribbean in collaboration with governments and partners. It focuses on actions and interventions within the context of gender and family support norms, stakeholder perceptions, and social inclusion considerations that are relevant to communicating risk and engaging communities to act. In Chap. 8, the authors discuss two national responses to COVID-19 in Latin America, specifically Chile and Paraguay, by exploring the cultural and trust dimensions in preventing and controlling transmission of the virus. The authors make an investment case for multi-dimensional, multimedia, and multi-audience approaches. Chapter 9 explores on-the-ground realities and challenges of responding to and managing a disease outbreak in an emergency/humanitarian setting. Emphasis is placed on the importance of interventions that are rights-based and informed by evidence.

Part III—Lessons Learned: Conclusions and Recommendations attempts to synthesize emerging themes from the case studies featured in Part II and their linkages to Part I (conceptual underpinnings). Moreover, we also put forward our own ideas with regard to the way forward, including practical recommendations for policy makers, donors, and practitioners involved in disease outbreak preparedness and response. Our main argument in Part III is that a holistic, systems-based, complex response to social science interventions is not yet fully implemented. While the case studies on various disease outbreaks that were covered in Part II provide sufficient practice-based evidence of applying multi-layered risk communication and community engagement strategies, not all these examples cover all six concepts put forward in this book to their full extent. Bio-medical advice underpinning risk communication based on what experts know about disease transmission at that point in time still dominates much of the work on communication. Compliance with behaviours to detect, isolate, treat, and stop transmission is driven more by epidemiological factors, hence leading to one-size-fits-all recommendations stemming from global guidance. Part III argues that without diluting the importance of bio-medical advice, a more systems view that takes into account risk communication and community engagement, culture, complexity, human rights, trust, and infodemics is needed. Without such a holistic approach, future outbreaks or pandemics will continue to face growing community resistance, distrust in responders and authorities, contribute to growing inequities, and further weaken preparedness and response strategies.

While the primary focus of this book and its collection of chapters is on expanding the range of concepts that can help strengthen pandemic and disease outbreak preparedness and response from a technical standpoint, we also acknowledge the inherent politicization of public health emergencies and disease outbreaks and fully recognize the importance of addressing the political dimensions of both preparedness and response efforts, as most recently experienced during the COVID-19 pandemic. The concepts discussed in the framework introduced in Chap. 1 recognize such political dimensions and their increasingly inherent presence in disease outbreak preparedness and response. As was noted at the beginning of this introduction, it is increasingly clear that addressing social, cultural, behavioural, and public dimensions of disease outbreak and pandemic preparedness and response needs a different level of attention to what may have been done up to now. More importantly, such attention needs to be a fluid and iterative effort, fully integrated into the regular work of public health systems, as opposed to the predominant one-off and reactive approach.

Through the following conceptual discussions and case studies we hope to contribute to the debate and, ideally, to the strengthening of the global architecture and national- and local-level responses. While perspectives about solutions put forward by each of the contributors may differ, the bottom line throughout the book remains clear. The world needs greater clarity and capacity to address the increasing challenges that infectious diseases pose not just to one country or a region, but often to humanity as a whole. The COVID-19 pandemic has indeed confirmed it. Whether it is a big or small outbreak, not to mention a pandemic, preparedness and response to disease outbreaks and pandemics must inevitably venture into and deal with the complexity of human behaviour and culture.

Las Vegas, NV, USA — Erma Manoncourt
Asunción, Paraguay — Rafael Obregon
Maputo, Mozambique — Ketan Chitnis

Contents

Contributors

Sharon Abramowitz, PhD Center for Global Health Science and Security, Georgetown University, Washington, DC, USA

Mohammad Alamgir, MPA Cox's Bazar Field Office, UNICEF Bangladesh, Cox's Bazar, Bangladesh

Ida-Marie Ameda, MSc Public Health, MSc Infectious Diseases Specialist in Emergencies, UNICEF ESARO, Nairobi, Kenya

Lawrence Sao Babawo, PhD School of Community Health Sciences, Njala University, Freetown, Sierra Leone

Jamie Bedson, MsocSc Independent Consultant, Seattle, WA, USA

Nayara Belle, MA Laboratorio de Geografia, Ambiente e Saude of the University of Brasilia, Brasília, Distrito Federal, Brazil

Aarunima Bhatnagar, MSc UNICEF, Baghdad, Iraq

Cox's Bazaar Field Office, UNICEF, Cox's Bazar, Bangladesh

Lotje Bijkerk, MSc Global Health The Netherlands Red Cross, The Hague, South-Holland, The Netherlands

Ketan Chitnis, PhD UNICEF Mozambique, Maputo, Mozambique

Julie Gerdes, PhD Technical and Professional Writing and Rhetoric, Department of English, Virginia Polytechnic Institute and State University, Blacksburg, VA, USA

Helen Gurgel, PhD Department of Geography, University of Brasilia, Brasília, Distrito Federal, Brazil

Mamunul Haque, MA, MDS UNICEF, Dhaka, Bangladesh

Sahar Hegazi, PhD UNICEF Regional Office for South Asia (ROSA), Amman, Jordan

Charles Kakaire, MPH (SBCC) UNICEF East and Southern Africa Regional Office (ESARO), Nairobi, Kenya

Foday Mahmoud Kamara, MPA Pandemic Preparedness Project, Njala University, Freetown, Sierra Leone

Neha Kapil, MSc UNICEF Middle East & North Africa Regional Office, Amman, Jordan

UNICEF Bangladesh, Dhaka, Bangladesh

Erma Manoncourt, PhD Management & Development Consulting, Inc., Las Vegas, NV, USA

Paolo Mefalopulos, PhD UNICEF, Santiago, Chile

Esther Yei Mokuwa, PhD Post-doctoral Fellow, Development Economics Group, Social Sciences, Wageningen University & Research, Wageningen, The Netherlands

Gelejimah Alfred Mokuwa, PhD Agricultural Sciences, Eastern Technical University, Kenema, Sierra Leone

Marion Baby-May Nyakoi, MSc Pandemic Preparedness Project, Njala University, Freetown, Sierra Leone

Rafael Obregon, PhD UNICEF, Asunción, Paraguay

Sam Oumo Okiror, MBChB, MPH Rapid Response Team, WHO Africa Region Office (AFRO), Brazzaville, Congo

Ataul Gani Osmani, MA Cox's Bazar Field Office, UNICEF, Cox's Bazar, Bangladesh

Eva Pilot, Dipl. Department of Health, Ethics and Society, Care and Public Health Research Institute (CAPHRI), Faculty of Health, Medicine and Life Sciences, Maastricht University, Maastricht, Limburg, The Netherlands

Sheikh Masudur Rahman, MSS UNICEF Dhaka, Dhaka, Bangladesh

Paul Richards, PhD Njala University, Freetown, Sierra Leone

Arianna Serino, MPH, MA Behavior Change and Community Health Advisor, Washington, DC, USA

About the Editors

Erma Manoncourt, PhD, is the Founder and President of Management & Development Consulting Inc., which provides technical support services to international development and humanitarian programmes, specializing in social and behaviour change programming and intervention design. She is an Adjunct Professor at the Paris School of International Affairs, Sciences Po in France, and Senior Lecturer at the New York University School of Global Public Health in the USA. Dr. Manoncourt is a Board member of the International Union of Health Promotion and Education (IUHPE) and Co-Chair of the IUHPE Global Working Group on the Social Determinants of Health. Most recently, she has provided technical support in Risk Communication and Community Engagement programming during both the Ebola Outbreak in West Africa (2014–2015) and the current COVID-19 pandemic.

Rafael Obregon, PhD, is the UNICEF Country Representative in Paraguay since July 2019. Prior to this, he led UNICEF's Communication for Development Section globally, was an Associate Professor at Ohio University, and worked as Regional Health Communication Specialist for the World Health Organization (WHO)/Pan American Health Organization (PAHO). He has supported several responses to humanitarian situations and to public health emergencies and disease outbreaks, including the 2014–2015 West Africa Ebola Outbreak and the 2016 Zika outbreak. He is a member of the Forum on Microbial Threats since 2017, and in 2016 served in the Advisory Committee to the WHO's International Health Regulations Emergency Committee on Zika virus. He has published extensively on global health communication and outbreak response.

Ketan Chitnis, PhD, is currently Chief of Communication for Development in UNICEF Mozambique. Previously he has worked with UNICEF in East-Asia and the Pacific Region and in New York. Ketan has worked on several disease outbreak responses since 2006 such as Avian and Pandemic Flu, Zika, Yellow Fever, Cholera, Ebola, and now COVID-19, supporting the UN's response for risk and behaviour change communication and community engagement. He has also worked on HIV/AIDS prevention, care and support, and on community health. He has taught and published on topics in communication for development and health communication in several journals.

Abbreviations

AAP	Accountability for Affected Populations
AAR	After-Action Review
BBCMA	BBC Media Action
BMGF	Bill and Melinda Gates Foundation
C4D	Communication for Development
CARPHA	The Caribbean Public Health Agency
CCE	Communication and Community Engagement
CDC	US Centers for Disease Control and Prevention
CE	Community Engagement
CEBS	Community Event-Based Surveillance
CFQs	Complaints, Feedback and Queries
CFR	Case Fatality Rate
CHW	Community Health Workers
CMVn	Community Mobilization Volunteer Network
cVDPV	Circulating Vaccine-Derived Poliovirus
CwC WG	Communicating with Communities Working Group
CXB	Cox's Bazaar
CZS	Congenital Zika Syndrome
DERCs	District Ebola Response Centres
DHMT	District Health Management Team
DRC	Democratic Republic of the Congo
EOC	Emergency Operations Center
ETC	Ebola Treatment Centre
EVD	Ebola Virus Disease
GBV	Gender-Based Violence
GPEI	Global Polio Eradication Initiative
HP	Hygiene Promoters
IEC	Information, Education and Communication
IFB	Islamic Foundation Bangladesh
IFCs	Information and Feedback Centre
IFRC	International Federation of Red Cross and Red Crescent Societies

IH	Information Hub
IHR	International Health Regulations
IPA	Innovations in Poverty Action
IPC	Interpersonal Communication
IPT	Interactive Participatory Theatre
IPV	Inactivated Polio Vaccine
ISIS	Islamic State in Iraq and Syria
ISP	Information Service Provider
JHU	Johns Hopkins University
JHU CCP	Johns Hopkins University Center for Communication Programs
KAP	Knowledge, Attitudes and Practice
LGBTQ	Lesbian, Gay, Bisexual, Transsexual, Queer
MERS	*Middle East Respiratory Syndrome*
MOH	Ministry of Health
MoI	Ministry of Information
MoRA	Ministry of Religious Affairs
NERC	National Ebola Response Centre
PCR	*Polymerase Chain Reaction*
PHEIC	Public Health Emergency of International Concern
PPE	Personal Protective Equipment
PSEA	Prevention of Sexual Exploitation and Abuse
RCCE	Risk Communication and Community Engagement
SARS	Severe Acute Respiratory Syndrome
SARS-CoV-2	Severe Acute Respiratory Syndrome Coronavirus 2
SMAC	Social Mobilization Action Committee
SOPs	Standard Operating Procedures
tOPV	Trivalent Oral Polio Vaccine
TWB	Translators Without Borders
UN	United Nations
USG	US Government
VHW	Village Health Worker
WHA	World Health Assembly
WHO	World Health Organization
ZAP	Zika AIRS Project
ZIKV	Zika Virus

Part I
Conceptual Framework

Chapter 1
Communication and Engagement in Disease Outbreaks and Pandemic Responses: Key Concepts and Issues

Rafael Obregon, Ketan Chitnis, and Erma Manoncourt

Contents

Introduction

Over the past 40 years, the world has confronted increasing infectious disease threats. While most of them remain as localized epidemics, restricted to certain geographic areas or countries, others increasingly turn into large scale outbreaks or pandemics (i.e., Cholera, HIV -Human Immunodeficiency Virus-, H1N1, and Severe acute respiratory syndrome coronavirus 2 - COVID-19 -) or into public health emergencies of international concern (i.e., Zika virus, Ebola Virus Disease - EVD). Globalization, international travel, trade, and many other factors have contributed to this shift in the behavior and potential multi-country and global impact of pathogens. In response to this trend, following a Workshop on Prioritization of Pathogens held in 2015, the World Health Organization (WHO) released a list of diseases "with potential to generate a public health emergency, and for which no, or insufficient, preventive and curative solutions exist" (p. 1). The list included diseases such as Lassa Fever, Ebola, Marburg, and emerging highly pathogenic

R. Obregon (✉)
UNICEF, Asunción, Paraguay
e-mail: robregon@unicef.org

K. Chitnis
UNICEF Mozambique, Maputo, Mozambique

E. Manoncourt
Management & Development Consulting, Inc., Las Vegas, NV, USA

E. Manoncourt et al. (eds.), *Communication and Community Engagement in Disease Outbreaks*, https://doi.org/10.1007/978-3-030-92296-2_1

coronaviruses such as Middle East Respiratory Syndrome (MERS) and Severe acute respiratory syndrome (SARS).

The aim of the WHO 2015 workshop was to accelerate research and development to "improve interventions and products such as diagnostics, vaccines, and therapeutics, behavioural interventions, and fill critical gaps in scientific knowledge to allow the design of better disease control measures" (WHO, 2015, p. 1) against those diseases. Just a few years later, since 2020, the COVID-19 pandemic has captured the international attention. And despite progress made in diagnostics and development of vaccines in record time, social and behavioral public health measures such as physical isolation and distancing, mask wearing, and handwashing remain at the center of efforts to bringing the virus under control and to returning to a reasonable level of normalcy which will certainly take significant time due to the emergence of new variants and evidence about the disease. Also, despite the unprecedented nature of COVID-19, the fact that it has become one of the most widespread disease outbreaks and pandemics in the past century —over 233 million confirmed cases as of September 2021, according to the Johns Hopkins University COVID-19 Resource Center—and that historically it is the third deadliest according to the WHO COVID-19 Dashboard, the reality is that several disease outbreaks and pandemics have occurred throughout the twentieth century (e.g., Spanish Flu, Asian Flu, Hong Kong Flu, HIV/AIDS). Furthermore, over the past 20 years, governments have responded to Swine Flu, SARS, MERS, and Avian Influenza outbreaks, and COVID-19 is, in fact, simply the most recent pandemic.

At the same time, globally the world is experiencing vector-borne communicable diseases such as Zika, Dengue, West Nile virus, and Chikungunya which have spread beyond original country borders due, to a large extent, to increased population mobility. Regular seasonal flu kills millions and seven different cholera outbreaks around the world have sickened many more. The most recent cholera pandemic occurred during the 1961–1975 period. It began in Indonesia (1961), spread across 24 countries in Asia, and eventually spread to 73 other countries in Africa, Europe, and the Americas (approximately 1.1 million cases reported globally) (Narkevich et al., 1993). In 1990, more than 90% of all cholera cases reported to WHO were from the African continent. Though the current cholera pandemic has affected some 120 countries, it largely remains a disease of impoverished, less-developed nations. For example, recent outbreaks occurred in Zimbabwe (2008–2009), Haiti (2010–2011) after an earthquake, as well as in Somalia and Yemen in 2017 in the context of internal conflict.

Over time, an increasing pattern of urbanization has become characteristic of disease outbreaks as well as the recognition that the globalization of disease has put both industrialized and low- and middle-income countries at risk. This warrants a global response that not only draws upon the golden standards of infectious disease response—detect, isolate, treat—but also upon factors such as the understanding of the social, psychological, and cultural dimensions of human behavior, for individuals, families, and communities. While this is not necessarily new and despite some progress in global efforts to strengthen the integration of social and behavioral factors in disease outbreak and pandemic response, broadening the scope of biomedical interventions to include a stronger focus on communication and engagement remains a considerable challenge for global and country-level organizations and for public health professionals.

This chapter, along with Chap. 2 (focused on community engagement principles and standards) and Chap. 3 (focused on how the global architecture of disease outbreak and pandemic response accommodate social and behavioral factors respectively), provides an overarching conceptual framework that sets the tone for the case studies featured in the second part of the book. In this chapter, we discuss key communication and engagement concepts and trends critical to preparedness and response to infectious disease outbreaks, epidemics, public health emergencies of international concern (PHEIC), and pandemics. We provide definitions of each concept, briefly illustrate the mportant role they have played in a wide range of outbreaks and pandemics, and highlight the increasing importance of addressing them in standard practice in infectious disease preparedness and response. While this cluster of concepts and trends is not exhaustive, we posit that they tend to regularly surface in most large disease outbreaks, epidemics, and pandemics, as it is illustrated throughout the case studies. Van Bavel et al. (2020) have taken a similar approach to discussing a variety of broader social and behavioral dynamics in the context of the COVID-19 response, while concepts such as syndemics (Singer et al., 2017; Mendenhall, 2015), which looks at the clustering of two or more epidemics, also put forward the importance of an eco-systemic approach to addressing the impact of disease.

A Brief Historical Perspective: Patterns, Behavioral Insights, Perceptions, and Understanding

The Ebola Virus Disease (EVD) Outbreak in West Africa (2014–2015) caused over 11,000 deaths, out of nearly 30,000 cases, and then occurred twice again in the Democratic Republic of the Congo (DRC) over the period 2019–2020: first, in the northeast part of the country (2287 deaths out of the 3324 confirmed cases) followed by a smaller outbreak in Equateur Province where 13 out of 18 health zones were affected, resulting in 55 deaths out of 130 confirmed cases.[1] The African experience shows that EVD tends to affect the most vulnerable communities in countries that already have high rates of poverty, face civil war or political unrest, and struggle with weak health systems and/or infrastructure. In both the West African and DRC outbreaks, a common characteristic is that EVD is no longer limited to rural areas, but it also affects marginalized communities in densely populated urban centers. Additionally, cross-border transmission was, and is, a worrisome factor that has further compounded an effective response given the limited availability of

[1] International Medical Corp. Democratic Republic of the Congo (DRC)—Ebola Situation Report #37—January 8, 2021.

public health resources. For example, the 2014–2015 outbreak reached other African countries and eventually Europe and the United States, and recent EVD outbreaks have threatened neighboring countries such as Uganda and Rwanda with cross-border transmission.

In all of those contexts, rumors, and misconceptions circulated widely due to public mistrust of messaging from formal government communication channels, access to different, alternate information sources, and confusion caused by competing, unclear information about what should be done. In West Africa, poor community linkages and poor health service quality undermined community perceptions and confidence, as well as the communities´ willingness to undertake, especially over long periods of time, preventive behaviors and other mitigating actions relevant to stopping the outbreak. As each of these recent outbreaks progressed, in a context of weak public health systems, engaging local communities in "bottoms-up" problem-solving was critical (Richards, 2016).

The emphasis of risk communication and community engagement (RCCE) approaches throughout the different epidemics and outbreaks, especially in their early phase, has often tended to focus on increasing risk perceptions among the population by underscoring the severity of disease and the vulnerability faced by different groups, followed by advising them on what to do. However, increasing efforts to raise awareness of the multiple factors that influence individual and collective behavior added to the recognition that, in addition to information and awareness, it was also important to address the social, behavioral, and communication dimensions affecting perceptions, beliefs, and practices. Several important behavioral insights and patterns have been learned about human behavior during different disease outbreaks, which include but are not limited to the following observations about public reactions and engagement:

- *Bystander effect: Reliance on others as "trusted sources" to determine the seriousness of a situation and diffused responsibility. There is a tendency for some to adopt a group mentality, which may involve following the behavior of individuals in their own social network or respected individuals from a wider reference group (*Darley & Latane, 1968).
- *New opinion leaders emerging as new sources of knowledge: For example, local community leaders in West Africa who convinced neighbors and family members to refrain from digging up their loved ones who have passed away to instead apply alternative burial rites that would still respect cultural norms, while maintaining the relevant disease prevention protocols.*
- *Bias toward normalcy: Responding to an emergency is outside of one's normal experience. It may be recalled that initially many considered that COVID-19 was simply like the seasonal flu, which did not warrant undue concern. In fact, it was observed that people may not react independently or be proactive but rather continue to wait and delay until instructions or more information are forthcoming.*
- *Selective perception and selective retention: Given the large amount of information disseminated, and sometimes conflicting statements made about the corona-*

virus and seasonal influenza, it has been noted that many in the public only focused on "facts" that fit their own world view and/or previous experience.

- *Emotional* vs. *rational thinking: A common tendency for many professionals is to assume that individuals are always rational in their choices and decision-making, but evidence also shows that in moments of crisis, especially high stress, they may act and react emotionally rather than logically. As such, their behavior may complicate an already difficult situation.*
- *Alarms are a single point of information—may not be enough to initiate a person or group into the expected emergency response: Behavior analysis shows that some did not take COVID-19 seriously until they or someone close to them have been affected. Even then, news articles surfaced describing individuals who were accessing information about Zika or Ebola from relatives living outside their infected communities. This was accomplished through their access to information on the internet and a wide range of social media channels.*
- *Psychological impact: A rising concern with COVID-19 confinements/lockdowns has been the emotional toll (*i.e., *stress, anxiety,* etc.*) that many individuals and their families' experience and stress due to the economic fallout of closed businesses and lack of employment, even if governments are providing subsidies which still may not be enough.*

Whereas a range of conspiracy theories have surfaced in polio endemic countries such as Pakistan and Afghanistan and in the context of the Ebola outbreaks in Africa, the volume of misinformation and disinformation has substantially increased as more outbreaks have occurred; one needs only to follow the public discourse during outbreaks of SARS and MERS to Ebola, Zika, and more recently COVID-19. These information challenges have been a predominant factor driving individual and collective behaviors and have thereby negatively impacted the effectiveness of mitigation and response efforts. As such, in addition to managing the disease outbreak itself, public health professionals must also contend with an "information epidemic" given multiple, conflicting information sources, and platforms. This has led to the establishment of a new practice discipline referred to as "infodemiology" and to the emergence of "infodemics," the concept that focuses on how rumors, disinformation, and misinformation impact the ecosystem of disease outbreaks and pandemic response.

The evolution of different disease outbreaks and pandemics and the increasing attention to social and behavioral dynamics have created and expanded the terminology being used to describe working with and engaging communities and the general public to achieve individual and/or social change that contributes to improved health outcomes. In the countries affected by Ebola, the terms "social mobilization" (SM), community engagement (CE), and the widely established term "communication for development" (C4D) were used almost inter-changeably by governments and global and local partners. Following WHO's adoption of the term risk communication and community engagement (RCCE) after the West Africa Ebola outbreak, its widespread use during the COVID-19 pandemic, and the increased attention to the power of risk perceptions in taking action, RCCE has become the common nomenclature currently being used to denote social and behavior change interventions that complement public information, political action, and government policies with the aim of engaging families, local communities, and the public at large.

As Claire Macdonald *at* Agence de Médecine Préventive summarized,[2] "preventing and controlling outbreaks is by no means an exact science." Macdonald points out that the West African Ebola outbreak showed how quickly a disease that had been relegated to "small outbreaks" could spin out of control. In fact, the past few years also have witnessed the rise of vaccine hesitancy as evidenced by an increasingly visible and vocal "anti-vaxxer" movement against regular childhood vaccinations in both Europe and North America. In 2021, the introduction of COVID-19 vaccines further complicated the situation and revealed how health literacy levels among a public in different cultural contexts can impact upon people´s understanding of the efficacy of different vaccine brands in protecting against the disease. The COVID-19 pandemic has further highlighted the difficulties in communicating real-time information to an initially skeptical public on a rapidly evolving virus that scientists were still learning about as it spread, caused diverse symptoms, and then mutated. This is not new either. In the case of cholera, for instance, in addition to poor access to health services, outbreaks have shown repeated patterns of human behavior that have contributed to ongoing periodic outbreaks despite multiple efforts to inform the public and to work with communities.

Disease outbreaks and pandemics are increasingly present in the public consciousness. As families and communities seek to understand what, when, and how to do and respond, there is a spillover effect in the political dimension as national and local governments react and attempt to respond. As such, the politicization of disease outbreaks, as experienced in West Africa during the Ebola outbreak, in Latin America during the Zika outbreak, and globally with COVID-19, has become a powerful factor that presents both a challenge and an opportunity for an effective public health response—essentially by setting the stage for interfacing human behavior and the science of epidemics and disease outbreaks. In short, the evolution of different disease outbreaks and pandemics, either vector-borne or caused by viruses or bacteria, has revealed over time the importance of addressing human behavior and engaging communities as a complement to the development of relevant and responsive social policies and the strengthening of health service delivery. These shifts, in turn, have led to the development and refinement of conceptual communication and engagement frameworks to guide effective prevention, mitigation, and response efforts.

[2] https://www.gavi.org/partnering-to-prevent-cholera-outbreaks-across

Toward a Communication and Engagement-Centered Conceptual Framework

As part of the support to governments and actors involved in public health emergencies, WHO and partners across the world have developed a wide range of tools and resources to operationalize how governments address pandemic, epidemic, and disease outbreak response. WHO (2020) outlines five stages for effective preparedness and response to infectious diseases: *anticipation, early detection, containment of the disease* at the early stages of transmission, *control and mitigation*, and the *elimination* of the risk of outbreak or *eradication* of the infectious disease (see Fig. 1.1). Each of these stages requires the implementation of interventions that include

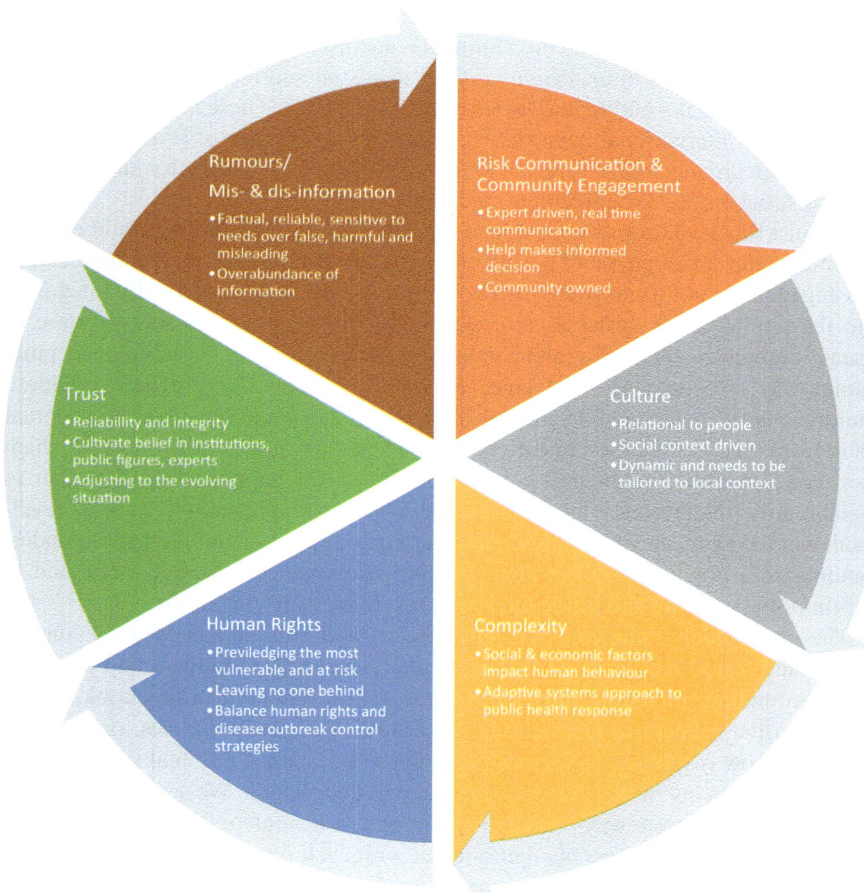

Fig. 1.1 A conceptual framework on communication and engagement for preparedness and response to disease outbreaks and pandemics

diagnostics, testing, contact tracing, quarantine, treatment and risk communication, and community engagement to achieve positive outcomes.

Risk communication, expanded to risk communication and community engagement (RCCE) after the West Africa 2014–2015 Ebola Outbreak, only gained greater focus and attention over the past few years after the recurring lessons learned from PHEIC such as Ebola and Zika. The reasons for this conceptual expansion stemmed not only from the transformations triggered by globalization of disease and other factors but also by the evolving dynamics of human behavior and global development and by the formulation of public health frameworks that are guided by principles and conventions centered on human rights, inclusion, and eco-systemic approaches that increasingly draw upon the social determinants of health. It has been widely documented, for instance, how engagement, dialogue, listening, and ownership became central to controlling the Ebola outbreak in West Africa (Richards, 2016; Abramowitz et al., 2014), while issues such as inclusion, in light of the emergence of stigma and discrimination against families and children affected by the Zika virus, and human rights related to sexual and reproductive health surfaced during the Zika outbreak (Davies & Bennett, 2016). These issues present new challenges to international agencies, governments, ministries of health, and other public health organizations responsible for or involved in preparing for and responding to disease outbreaks, epidemics, and pandemics.

Against this backdrop, we introduce six concepts that we believe could eventually inform the development of a conceptual framework centered on communication and engagement to further strengthen how these issues are systematically integrated into the public health systems and, specifically, in preparedness and response to disease outbreaks, epidemics, and pandemics. Jabareen (2009) defines a conceptual framework "as a network, or 'plane,' of linked concepts that together provide a comprehensive understanding of a phenomenon." Jabareen adds that "conceptual frameworks are not merely collections of concepts but, rather, constructs in which each concept plays an integral role…and provide an interpretative approach to social reality." Numerous conceptual frameworks in public health have been developed over the years, most of which tend not only to provide a comprehensive understanding of a phenomenon but also to guide empirical and applied work and to inform policy making and guide interventions (Solar & Irwin, 2010).

The conceptual framework we put forward will certainly need to be further refined and tested but we hope that given its conceptual, empirical, and practice-based grounding, including through the case studies featured in this book, it will trigger further reflections and actions. The COVID-19 pandemic has, once again, illustrated how responses to various pandemics and disease outbreaks approached and dealt with many of the concepts discussed in this chapter. We argue that this has been done in a discrete way—each concept seen as a single unit—as opposed to a complementary set of concepts that interact with each other even if in some cases they may overlap. Arguably, for instance, a primary focus on risk communication drove the early phase of the COVID-19 response, while discussions about human rights have remained, at least in the early phase, peripheral. While key biomedical principles of disease outbreak and pandemic preparedness and response should remain as the driving force, a broader perspective that draws on eco-systemic frameworks, in this case through the communication and engagement lens, will add great value to the implementation of people-centered approaches.

The first concept we introduce is ***risk communication and community engagement***. As discussed in the Introduction to this book and in Chapter 3, risk communication was one of the core capacity areas included in the IHR released in 2005. WHO (2005) states that risk communication is the "exchange of real-time information, advice and opinions between experts and people facing threats to their health, economic or social well-being, and that the ultimate purpose of risk communication is to enable people at risk to make informed decisions to protect themselves and their loved ones." Similarly, community engagement focuses on the role that community stakeholders, including individuals and community members, play in responding to an outbreak and on their ownership of the response. In many ways, risk and communication and community engagement are two sides of the same coin.

As a result of lessons learned from the 2014–2015 Ebola outbreak, it was clear that the focus on risk communication was not sufficient to ensure community ownership and involvement in preparedness and response. Arguably, only after the 2014–2015 Ebola outbreak in West Africa did community engagement generate the type of attention it has today within global and country decision making bodies in public health. While cultural practices, rituals, and related norms and behaviors have been addressed in health communication efforts for decades (from promotion of family planning to HIV prevention to polio eradication), the challenge posed by Ebola in West Africa eventually pushed decision-makers and international health experts and local teams to broaden efforts to engage communities in the response. Thus, during and after the Ebola outbreak of 2014–2015, risk communication and community engagement gradually became a critical function and an integral pillar of the WHO outbreak response framework (WHO, 2018).

Risk communication and community engagement as a core pillar of disease outbreak preparedness and response must be operational, in principle, as soon as the EOC (emergency operation center) has been activated in the context of a public health emergency. The integration of risk communication and community engagement as complementary component is now well reflected in global guidance and tools developed by agencies such as WHO, UNICEF, and the International Federation of the Red Cross (IFRC). While this has been an important development, the effective integration and implementation of risk communication and community engagement continues to face important challenges, especially at country level, to a large extent due to the tendency to implement them as two separate areas of work or to prioritize the communication of risk, as well as to the limited focus and resourcing that ministries of health often give to this component.

The second concept we introduce is ***culture***. While the role of culture in development has been the subject of heated debates and analysis, it has also been discussed widely in the context of public health. McMullin and Rushing (2018) refer to it as "a complex system of meanings...relational and learned...and as a dynamic process of meaning making that is informed and constrained by social contexts." They add that "as a shared meaning system, culture includes conscious and unconscious assumptions and it assists in the interpretation of individual experience and guides future expectations and actions." Importantly, these dimensions regularly inform how individuals, groups and economics engage in specific behaviors relevant to public health issues.

The role of culture in disease prevention and control, including in pandemic and disease outbreak preparedness and response, however, is not a new topic. Several authors have discussed how greater attention to cultural dimensions can enhance effective public health interventions, including communication interventions (Van Bavel et al., 2020; Kreuter & McClure, 2004; Olofuwote & Aranda, 2018; Airhihenbuwa, 1995). Cultural dimensions in HIV prevention, for instance, played a critical role (and continue to) both to engage key stakeholders and affected communities in promotion and uptake of preventative behaviors (McKee, Bertrand and Becker-Benton 2004) and to address stigmatization and discrimination (Raman, 2013) in the HIV response. The use of culturally appropriate messages and culturally sensitive communication have become standard guidance for planners and implementers, while more critical perspectives have pushed for culture-centered and participatory approaches in which affected communities could have a more prominent role in determining the type and focus of public health interventions (Dutta, 2008).

Yet, as several authors also have argued, the integration of culture in public health still shows important gaps. Kreuter and McClure (2004) make this point very forcefully:

> Although culture is widely accepted as a factor associated with health and behavior, its role in public health practice and research to date has been more rhetorical than applied. For example, while terms like cultural sensitivity and cultural appropriateness are now standard in the parlance of public health professionals, operational definitions, measures, and explanatory models of culture and health are lacking (p. 440).

The third concept we introduce is ***complexity***, especially as they relate to the role of social and behavioral determinants. One of the most important conceptual shifts in public health over the past few decades has been the increasing emphasis on the social determinants of health, particularly on how health inequalities are not just dependent upon the behaviors of individuals and communities but also upon how social and economic factors and drivers determine the way people behave as well as their health status and wellbeing (Marmot & Wilkinson, 2006). Taft and Bandyopadhyay (2011) have taken this notion to another level by linking public health systems, and by extension how they respond to disease outbreaks and epidemics, to complex adaptive systems. They argue that:

> *An increasing emphasis on the social determinants of health, a more complicated technological and global world and an understanding that human societies can be conceived as complex adaptive systems, have led public health scholars to take an interest in the science of complexity. Complexity science has been described as the study of complex adaptive systems to see 'the patterns of relationships within them, how they are sustained, how they self-organize and how outcomes emerge' ([1], p. 3). National or local communities, community health services, general practices and public hospitals embedded in political,*

economic and cultural contexts all act as complex adaptive systems and shape the behaviors of health care professionals, citizens and patients in sometimes unpredictable ways.

More importantly, Taft and Bandyopadhyay posit that modern public health requires exploring new approaches and solutions to effectively address an increasingly complex socio-economic environment and context. Arguably, disease outbreak response and preparedness are, by definition, and especially in an increasingly globalized world, significantly complex and require appropriate responses. The need to address social and behavioral determinants along with the demands of the fast-paced environments we live in, especially due to the rapid development of communication technologies, pose considerable challenges to decision makers. This reality has not gone unnoticed to researchers involved in the application of complexity science to disease outbreak preparedness and response. Pourbholoul et al. (2018) have put forward practical recommendations to apply elements of complexity to this area of work including elements that look at behavioral issues such as network analysis and the identification of personal contacts in outbreak settings.

The fourth concept we introduce is ***human rights***. The increasing number of widespread epidemics and PHEIC as well as pandemics such as the COVID-19 over the past few years has put human rights squarely at the center of preparedness and response efforts. While human rights-based approaches to development and emergency response have been integrated into international development frameworks since the late 1990s, the implementation of strict measures such as quarantine, social and physical isolation, physical distance, lockdowns, and school closures, amongst others, are often framed as impinging upon people's fundamental rights to movement, participation, leisure, worship, and work, to name a few (Rollison, 2015). How to balance restrictive public health measures with the ability to exercise fundamental rights has become increasingly challenging both for public health authorities and communities.

While there are principles and protocols adopted by the United Nations and the WHO that may guide countries to impose state of emergencies and in turn to restrict freedom of movement in the broader interest of public health, these measures must be lawful and consider the disproportionate impact of restrictions on people, especially upon the most vulnerable and marginalized groups. Human rights organizations argue that even if certain rights are suspended for public health reasons, freedom of expression including the right to seek and disseminate information needs to be protected as per international law (Human Rights Watch, 2020). Yet, in several recent outbreaks human rights have come to odds with the response to public health emergencies, especially PHEICs such as Ebola, Zika, and COVID-19.

Smith (2006), for instance, has argued that "many of the public health measures used during the SARS outbreaks, especially isolation and quarantine, may conflict with certain human rights. In order to plan a response to global infectious disease outbreaks it will therefore be important to consider a range of issues concerning the nexus between containment and human freedoms." Amnesty International (2020) has documented how the response to epidemics and disease outbreaks may intersect with various human rights including in the case of the recent COVID-19 pandemic.

The fundamental challenge is how to ensure that effective protection measures such as quarantine and social isolation are implemented within the confines of protection of people's human rights, for which communication and engagement is critical. Rather than going away, this issue is likely to arise more frequently in future responses to outbreaks and pandemics, therefore it needs specific consideration in pandemic preparedness and response.

The fifth concept we introduce is ***trust***. While all the concepts discussed previously are crucial to effective disease outbreak preparedness and response, *Trust* has emerged, perhaps, as the bedrock upon which other interventions, biomedical or of the types discussed in this book, rest and depend upon for effective implementation (Forum on Microbial Threats, 2017). UNICEF and the IFRC (2020) have defined trust in emergency response as "a firm belief in the reliability and integrity of a person or institution. It is critical currency for health emergency preparedness and response, which relies on the whole of society buy-in and cooperation" (p. 6). Trust operates at different levels: community trust in government authorities and healthcare systems, trust of community members and individuals in healthcare providers, and public trust in media and communication sources and channels, among others (Olonge et al., 2019).

Various studies validate this point. Low levels of trust often can have a significant negative impact on different components of preparedness and response, from case detection to contact tracing to seeking treatment early to engaging in preventive behaviors (Winck et al., 2019). An empirical study conducted by Winck and colleagues, for instance, reported a correlation between trust in government and compliance with government EVD control measures during the Ebola outbreak response in North Kivu in 2019. Also, the experience of polio eradication in several countries shows how building trust at different levels—with communities, among communities, in health providers, and in the government—was critical to achieving the desired goal (Solomon, 2019; Stamidis et al., 2019; SteelFisher et al., 2015; Obregon & Waisbord, 2010).

The sixth and last concept we introduce is ***rumors, disinformation, and misinformation***. While these issues are not new to the dynamics of public health emergencies and disease outbreaks, the rapid growth of social media and its convergence with news media has catapulted information and communication to the forefront (Kou et al., 2017). Concepts such as disinformation, defined as "false, harmful and misleading content in media and information ecosystems" (OECD, 2020), and "infodemics", defined as "an overabundance of information—some accurate and some not—that makes it hard for people to find trustworthy sources and reliable guidance when they need it" (PAHO, 2020), have attempted to capture the extent to which rumors and false information have influenced public perceptions and behaviors related to public health emergencies and disease outbreaks, as well as the actual response that governments and authorities have mounted to address these challenges (Islam et al., 2020; Roberts, 2017).

Numerous studies have both documented well and provided strong empirical evidence of the role of rumors and misinformation in the implementation of public health initiatives and actions, especially those related to response to pandemics and infectious disease outbreaks (Kirk Sell, Hosangadi and Trotochaud, 2020; Ghenai & Mejova, 2017). A study by Gallotti et al. (2020) "found that measurable waves of potentially unreliable information preceded the rise of Covid-19 infections, exposing entire countries to falsehoods that pose a serious threat to public health" (p. 1285). Based on the existing and growing evidence, we believe that one of the most important trends and realities in pandemic and disease outbreak response is that rumors, disinformation, and misinformation have become part and parcel of their landscape. This, in turn, means that the public health community has limited or no alternative but to regularly take this dimension—rumors and misinformation—into account across preparedness and response efforts and assess the extent to which it interfaces with other key concepts discussed in this chapter.

While each of these concepts could be addressed and analyzed independently of each other, and in fact that is how it has been done thus far, we believe that due to their organic interaction, which is manifested in the daily lives of individuals and communities, its integrated analysis and deliberate integration into public health systems and into preparedness and response approaches is critical to strengthening how global and country level public health institutions and organizations address these issues. As Fig. 1.1 shows, for instance, community engagement is integral to building trust and vice versa. Similarly, the tensions that may arise from perceived restrictions to the exercise of basic rights requires substantive communication and engagement, while rumors, disinformation, and misinformation can have substantive negative impacts on trust-building.

If the proposed conceptual framework, with the empirical and practice-based support that the case studies provide, makes sense, then the next question is how a framework like the one we put forward in this chapter can best contribute to improving disease outbreak and epidemic and pandemic preparedness and response. The global architecture of the disease outbreak and pandemic response, discussed in more detail and through the lens of the Zika outbreak and the COVID-19 pandemic in Chap. 3, is critical to facilitate the integration of the earlier concepts into global and country-level approaches. The IHR initiatives such as One Health, an interdisciplinary approach to holistically look at the interface between humans, animals and eco-systems within which we operate as the crucible of new and emerging infectious diseases (Calistri et al., 2013), and operational mechanisms such as the global risk communication and community engagement collective co-led by global health and development organizations involved in disease outbreak and pandemic response (IFRC, 2020) provide interesting options to test and refine this framework.

This expanded scope of a communication and engagement-centered approach that complements the standard biomedical response to disease outbreak and epidemic and pandemic preparedness and response should also be a recognition of the interdependence of social science and medicine. It was during the West Africa Ebola outbreak that greater attention was paid to rapid, localized, social, and medical anthropological insights combined with communication and community capacities related to behaviors such as burials and caregiving at home, which initially were critical drivers of transmission. These drivers of transmission in turn became a priority and complemented infection prevention and control measures in primary health centers or Ebola treatment centers. Likewise, perception, trust, and interpersonal communication between communities and health workers has been found to have great influence upon early detection and prevention of Ebola transmission and upon greater care seeking practices, rather than the sole reliance on surveillance and clinical care. Experience has also shown that effective contact tracing depends heavily upon the extent to which communities trust the responders and the presence of rapport that is based on open and transparent communication, as in the case of the Ebola outbreak in North Kivu, DRC in 2018–2019. This is also the case with polio vaccination teams in South Asia and parts of Africa (Stamidis, 2019; Ghinai, 2013; Obregon & Waisbord, 2010). By 2021, in the context of the COVID-19 pandemic, not only is the central role of communication and engagement more evident and unquestionable, but there is also an urgent need to understand how concepts and issues included in this framework interact with each other in order to guide more effective preparedness and response.

Disclaimer The views expressed in this chapter are those of the authors and do not represent the official position of UNICEF.

References

Abramowitz, S., Hipgrave, D., Witchard, A., & Heyman, D. (2014). Lessons from the West Africa Ebola epidemic: A systematic review of epidemiological and social and behavioral science research priorities. *Journal of Infectious Diseases, 218*(11), 1730–1738.

Airhihenbuwa, C. (1995). *Health and culture: Beyond the Western paradigm*. Sage.

Amnesty International (2020). Coivd-19 Pandemic: Human Rights in times of Crisis. V12, 50. https://www.amnesty.ca/blog/covid-19-pandemic-human-rights-times-crises.

Calistri, P., Iannetti, S., Danzetta, M., Narcisi, V., Cito, F., Di Sabatino, D., Bruno, R., Sauro, F., Atzeni, M., Carvelli, A., & Giovannini, A. (2013). The components of 'one world – one health' approach. *Transboundary and Emerging Diseases, 60*(Suppl 2), 4–13. https://doi.org/10.1111/tbed.12145

Darley, J. M., & Latane, B. (1968). Bystander intervention in emergencies: Diffusion of responsibility. *Journal of Personality and Social Psychology, 8*(4 Pt 1), 377–383. https://doi.org/10.1037/h0025589

Davies, S., & Bennett, B. (2016). A gendered human rights analysis of Ebola and Zika: Locating gender in global health emergencies. *International Affairs, 92*(5), 1041–1060. https://doi.org/10.1111/1468-2346.12704

Day, M. (2016). Human-animal health interactions: The role of one health. *American Family Physician, 93*(5), 344–346.

Dutta, M. 2008. Communicating health: A culture-centered approach. Polity.

Forum on Microbial Threats. (2017). Building communication capacity to counter infectious disease threats: Proceedings of a workshop. In *National academies of sciences, engineering, and medicine, health and medicine division, board on global health*. Forum on Microbial Threats National Academies Press.

Gallotti, R., Valle, F., Castaldo, N., Saco, P., & De Domenico, M. (2020). Assessing the risks of 'infodemics' in response to COVID-19 epidemics. *Nature Human Behavior, 4*, 1285–1293.

Ghenai, A. and Y. Mejova. 2017."Catching Zika Fever: Application of Crowdsourcing and Machine Learning for Tracking Health Misinformation on Twitter." arXiv preprint arXiv:1707.03778. arxiv.org.

Ghinai, I., Willott, C., Dadari, I., & Larson, H. (2013). Listening to the rumours: What the northern Nigeria polio vaccine boycott can tell us ten years on. *Global Public Health., 8*(10), 1138–1150. https://doi.org/10.1080/17441692.2013.859720

Human Rights International (2020). "Human rights dimensions of the Covid-19 response". March 19. Human Rights Dimensions of COVID-19 Response I Human Rights Watch (hrw.org) (accessed on September 30 2021).

Jabareen, Y. (2009). Building a conceptual framework: Philosophy, definitions and procedures. *International Journal of Qualitative Methods, 8*(4), 49–62.

Khan, Y., O'Sullivan, T., Brown, A., et al. (2018). Public health emergency preparedness: A framework to promote resilience. *BMC Public Health, 18*, 1344. https://doi.org/10.1186/s12889-018-6250-7

Kirk Sell, T., Hosangadi, D., & Trotochaud, M. (2020). Misinformation and the US Ebola communication crisis: Analyzing the veracity and content of social media messages related to a fear-inducing infectious disease outbreak. *BMC Public Health, 20*, 550. https://doi.org/10.1186/s12889-020-08697-3

Kreuter, M., & McClure, S. (2004). The role of culture in health communication. *The Annual Review of Public Health, 24*, 439–455. https://doi.org/10.1146/annurev.publhealth.25.101802.123000

Marmot, M., & Wilkinson, R. G. (Eds.). (2006). *Social determinants of health* (2nd ed.). Oxford University Press.

McKee, N., Bertrand, J., & Becker-Benton, A. (2004). *Strategic communication in the HIV/AIDS epidemic*. Sage.

McMullin, J., & Rushing, S. (2018). Culture and public health. In *Oxford bibliographies*. Oxford University Press. https://doi.org/10.1093/OBO/9780199756797-0009

Mendenhall, E. (2015). Bbeyond comorbidity: A critical perspective of syndemic depression and diabetes in cross-cultural contexts. *Medical Anthropology Quarterly, 30*, 462–478.

Narkevich, M., Onischenko, G., Lomov, J., Moskvitina, E., Podosinnikova, L., & Medinsky, G. (1993). The seventh pandemic of cholera in the USSR, 1961-89. *Bulletin of the World Health Organization, 71*(2), 189–196. PMC 2393457. PMID 8490982.

Obregon, R., & Waisbord, S. (2010). ˝the complexity of social mobilization in health communication: Top-down and bottom-up experiences in polio eradication˝. *Journal of Health Communication., 15*(supplement 1), 25–47.

Olofuwote, J., & Aranda, J. (2018). The PEN-3 cultural model: A critical review of health communication for Africans and African immigrants. In Y. Mao & R. Ahmed (Eds.), *Culture, migration, and health communication in a global context* (pp. 177–190). Routledge.

Organisation for Economic Co-operation and Development (OECD). (2020). *Transparency, communication and trust: The role of public communication in responding to the wave of disinformation about the new coronavirus*. Retrieved from http://www.oecd.org/coronavirus/policy-responses/transparency-communication-and-trust-bef7ad6e/

Pan American Health Organization. (2020). *Understanding the Infodemic and misinformation in the fight against COVID-19*. Retrieved April 30, 2021, from https://iris.paho.org/handle/10665.2/52052.

Pourbohloul, B., English, K., & Hupert, N. (2018). Complexity, the bridging science of emerging respiratory outbreak response. In E. Mitleton-Kelly (Ed.), *Handbook of research methods in complexity science* (pp. 327–355). Elgar Publishing.

Richards, P. (2016). *Ebola: How a people's science helped end an epidemic (African arguments)*. Zedbooks.

Rollison, R. (2015). "Human rights in the era of epidemics". Advocates Forum, pp. 47–55. University of Chicago. https://crownschool.uchicago.edu/public-health-and-human-rights-era-epidemics

Singer, M., Bulled, N., Ostrach, B., & Mendenhall, E. (2017). Syndemics and the biosocial conception of health. *The Lancet, 389*, 941–950.

Smith, R. (2006). Responding to global infectious disease outbreaks: Lessons from SARS on the role of risk perception, communication and management. *Social Science Medicine, 63*(12), 3113–3123. https://doi.org/10.1016/j.socscimed.2006.08.004
Solar, O., & Irwin, A. (2010). *A conceptual framework for action on the social determinants of health.* Discussion Paper. WHO Document Production Services.
Solomon, R. (2019). Involvement of civil society in India's polio eradication program: Lessons learned. *American Journal of Tropical Medicine and Hygiene., 101*(supplement 4), 15–20. https://doi.org/10.4269/ajtmh.18-0931
Stamidis, K., et al. (2019). Trust, communication, and community networks: How the CORE Group polio project community volunteers led the fight against polio in Ethiopia's Most at-risk areas. *American Journal of Tropical Medicine and Hygiene., 101*(supplement 4), 59–67. https://doi.org/10.4269/ajtmh.19-0038
SteelFisher, G., Blendon, R., Guirguis, S., et al. (2015). Threats to polio eradication Pakistan and Nigeria: A polling study of caregivers of children younger than 5 years. *The Lancet-Infectious Diseases, 15*(10), 1183–1192.
Stellmach, D., Beshar, I., Bedford, J., Du Cross, P., & Stringer, B. (2018). Anthropology in public health emergencies: What is anthropology good for? *BMJ Global Health, 2018*(3), e000534.
Taft, A., & Bandyopadhyay, M. (2011). Introduction to COMPASS: Navigating complexity in public health research. *BMC Public Health, 11*(5), 1–3.
United Nations Children's Fund (UNICEF)/International Federation of Red Cross Societies (IFRC). (2020). *Building Trust Within and Across Communities for Health Emergency Preparedness.* Retrieved from https://apps.who.int/gpmb/assets/thematic_papers_2020/tp_2020_3.pdf
Van Bavel, J., et al. (2020). Using social and behavioral science to support COVID-19 pandemic response. *Nature Human Behavior, 4*(5), 460–471. https://doi.org/10.1038/s41562-020-0884-z
World Health Organization (WHO). (2005). *EURO IHR core capacities.* Retrieved February 28, 2021, from https://www.euro.who.int/en/health-topics/health-emergencies/international-health-regulations/capacity-building/ihr-core-capacities
World Health Organization (WHO). (2015). *Blueprint for R&D preparedness and response to public health emergencies due to highly infectious pathogens.* World Health Organization.
World Health Organization. (2018). *Risk Communication and Community Engagement (RCCE) Considerations: Ebola Response in the Democratic Republic of the Congo.* World Health Organization.
World Health Organization (WHO). (2020). *Operational planning guidelines to support country preparedness and response.* World Health Organization.
World Health Organization (WHO). (2021). *Global Covid-19 Dashboard, as of February 2021.*

Chapter 2
The Global Health Architecture of Pandemic Preparedness and Response: Comparing and Contrasting Experiences of Zika and COVID-19 in Brazil

Lotje Bijkerk, Nayara Belle, Helen Gurgel, and Eva Pilot

Contents

Background

Introduction

In human history, numerous infectious diseases resulted in high death tolls, panic, and economic and political instability. The current COVID-19 pandemic shows the global public health system's frailty and the urgent need to strengthen preparedness and response to Public Health Emergencies of International Concern (PHEIC). Global, national, and local responses to COVID-19 and future PHEICs can be improved when looking back and learning from the strengths and weaknesses of

L. Bijkerk
Maastricht University, Maastricht, Limburg, The Netherlands

Universidade de Brasília, Brasília, Distrito Federal, Brazil

N. Belle · H. Gurgel
Universidade de Brasília, Brasília, Distrito Federal, Brazil

E. Pilot (✉)
Maastricht University, Maastricht, Limburg, The Netherlands
e-mail: eva.pilot@maastrichtuniversity.nl

E. Manoncourt et al. (eds.), *Communication and Community Engagement in Disease Outbreaks*, https://doi.org/10.1007/978-3-030-92296-2_2

responses of past PHEICs. The present chapter is based on an original research conducted between November 2019 and July 2020 in a collaboration between Maastricht University and Universidade de Brasília. Our study aimed to give an overview of the lessons learned from the responses to Zika virus (ZIKV)[1] and COVID-19 PHEIC and the recommendations given by experts, based on their experiences, insights, and opinions. The responses to ZIKV were compared and contrasted to the current responses to the COVID-19 pandemic. This research focused on risk communication, (global) politics and framing, and structural problems, including (gender-)inequality, during the ZIKV PHEIC and the COVID-19 pandemic. Based on the lessons learned, we discuss recommendations on how the global health architecture—explained in the next section—can enhance its capability to effectively prepare and respond as an international community to the increasing threat of worldwide (re-)emerging diseases. As we will discuss throughout this chapter, strengthening the risk communication and community engagement components within the global health architecture is needed to enhance these aspects during public health emergencies.

We start this chapter with an overview of the elements of global health architecture. We will then discuss the results of our study, comparing and contrasting the preparedness and response actions to the ZIKV and COVID-19 PHEICs, and give an overview of the lessons learned. Based on these lessons, we formulated recommendations on improving the global health architecture, focusing on reflections about risk communication and community engagement.

The Global Health Architecture in Public Health Emergencies

Cooperation between states to prevent the international spread of infectious diseases started in the mid-nineteenth century when the International Sanitary Conferences were held to standardize international quarantine regulations. When the WHO evolved in 1948, it revised the International Sanitary Regulations extensively and adopted the International Health Regulations (IHR) in 1969 (Howard-Jones, 1975). The outbreaks and rapid spread of severe acute respiratory syndrome (SARS) in 2003 highlighted constraints of the IHR 1969 (Merianos & Peiris, 2005). Acknowledging the fact that the risk of new and re-emerging infectious diseases was growing every year, the IHR 1969 were extensively revised. In 2005, the new IHR were adopted, featuring strategies to cope with unknown risks of an interconnected world (Fidler & Gostin, 2006). Furthermore, the focus shifted from commercial interests (travel and trade) to public health protection (Fidler, 2005). The IHR is a reaction to the need for global efforts to detect and contain epidemics and legally bind 196 countries to strengthen

[1] In this chapter, we use the scientific abbreviation ZIKV for the more common names "Zika" or "Zika virus."

epidemics' global control efforts and stimulate working together for global health security. The IHR aim to prevent, protect, and control the international spread of disease in a way that avoids unnecessary interference with international traffic and trade (WHO, 2016a). The IHR contain 13 core capacities, including risk communication (WHO, 2021). Effective risk communication is crucial for managing public health emergencies in an interconnected world (Nuttall & Odugleh-Kolev, 2012).

Under the IHR, the WHO can declare a (threat of a) disease outbreak a Public Health Emergency of International Concern (PHEIC). To be considered a PHEIC, an outbreak must pose public health risks beyond the affected country and be severe enough to require a coordinated international response. The declaration requires a final decision of the Director-General of the WHO, relying on a roster of experts appointed as Emergency Committee, advising and recommending public health interventions (WHO, 2016a). After the declaration of a PHEIC, countries are obliged to respond adequately, and solidarity should evoke, as well as international cooperation, fastened scientific research and international support to affected countries (Bedford et al., 2020; Fischer & Katz, 2010). Since the entrance of the IHR 2005, six PHEICs were declared: the H1N1 influenza virus pandemic in 2009; the resurgence of wild poliovirus in 2014; the West Africa Ebola virus epidemic in 2014; the Zika virus (ZIKV) epidemic in 2016; the Kivu Ebola epidemic in 2019; and the current COVID-19 pandemic (2020) (Giesecke & STAG-IH, 2019; WHO 2020a, b).

The WHO, the IHR, the Emergency Committees, and the PHEIC form the base of the global health architecture discussed in this chapter.

ZIKV and COVID-19 as PHEICs: A Brief Overview

In 2016, the ZIKV epidemic in Brazil was declared a PHEIC. ZIKV is a vector-borne disease that is primarily and quickly transmitted via *Aedes aegypti* mosquitos but also perinatally, sexually and via transfusion (Bueno, 2017; Epelboin et al., 2017; Musso et al., 2015). By the end of 2014, an unknown dengue-like disease outbreak, later confirmed ZIKV, was reported in Northeastern Brazil (Avelino-Silva & Kallas, 2018; Possas, 2016; Zanluca et al., 2015). Concurrently, there was a significant increase in Guillain–Barré syndrome cases and other neurological defects, and dramatic growth in the number of babies born with microcephaly and other congenital malfunctions (Chang et al., 2016; Lowe et al., 2018; Oliveira et al., 2017). Since ZIKV also spread outside Brazil, it was viewed as an international threat to public health. The Director-General of the WHO declared ZIKV and the possible association with neurological disorders and congenital malformations as a PHEIC on February 1, 2016. The Emergency Committee's advice to declare a PHEIC was based on the high possibility of association, but lack of an established causal link (Heymann et al., 2016). Extensive case–control studies confirmed the link between microcephaly and

ZIKV infection during pregnancy (Brady et al., 2019; Brasil et al., 2016; de Araújo et al., 2016). It became clear that ZIKV infection during pregnancy was not only associated with microcephaly, but with a wide range of congenital malformations and neurological disorders, grouped in the term Congenital Zika syndrome (CZS) (Brasil et al., 2016; Jamrozik & Selgelid, 2018; Kuper et al., 2019; van der Linden et al., 2016). Following sufficient evidence for a causal link and further understanding of the consequences of the ZIKV outbreak, the Emergency Committee decided on November 18, 2016, that ZIKV and associated consequences did no longer represent a PHEIC as defined under the IHR (WHO, 2016b). By the end of 2019, there were 3474 confirmed cases of children affected by CZS in Brazil, although there is a great possibility that there are many more children affected, but not officially diagnosed (Fraser & Alves, 2019; Ministério da Saúde, 2019).

Currently, we see that (re-)emerging infectious diseases continue to pose threats to global health. On January 30, 2020, the WHO declared a new PHEIC: the outbreak of novel coronavirus (SARS-CoV-2) which causes the coronavirus disease 2019 (COVID-19) (WHO, 2020a). The first infected cases were detected in December 2019 in Wuhan, China, from where it spread to 190 countries and regions. On June 5, 2021, there are over 172.6 million global confirmed cases and 3.7 million global deaths, from which Brazil has the third-highest number in cases (over 16.8 million) and second in deaths (over 470,000) (JHU, 2021). As with ZIKV, the COVID-19 pandemic shows challenges with evidence-based decision-making, sustainable solutions, and widening socio-economic and gender inequalities. The COVID-19 pandemic, therefore, shows once again the frailty of the global public health system and the urgent need to strengthen epidemic and pandemic responses.

Lessons from the PHEIC of ZIKV and the COVID-19 Pandemic for the Global Health Architecture

In the following section, we discuss the main lessons learned and recommendations during the ZIKV outbreak in Brazil based on the experiences and opinions of 13 experts (Table 2.1) and additional literature research. A reflection on the current COVID-19 pandemic response is provided for each topic, comparing and contrasting it to the ZIKV PHEIC. An overview can be found in Box 2.1. The results are based on (online) in-depth qualitative interviews with seven experts and a qualitative survey, completed by six experts. Participants' survey answers and interviews were linked to ID numbers (ID1, ID2, …) and will be used as references in the following section.

Box 2.1 Main lessons learned of the responses to the PHEIC of ZIKV, with reflections on the responses to the COVID-19 PHEIC

Communication and uncertainty: Uncertainty played a main role in the ZIKV crisis since the PHEIC was declared because of the uncertainty surrounding the association between microcephaly and ZIKV. The ZIKV responses showed that effective public awareness, risk communication, coordination, and transparency are essential and that rational policies should be formulated rather than policies driven by fear and uncertainty. The chaotic and contradictive messages of the current Brazilian government in the COVID-19 PHEIC show that the lessons learned in ZIKV about risk communication and uncertainty still pose significant challenges.

Preparedness and surveillance: The ZIKV PHEIC showed that a strong surveillance system and public health structure are crucial in notifying and reacting adequately to a PHEIC. It also brought to the fore, once again, that investing in preparedness rather than predominantly investing in response once the crisis arrives is very political, yet crucial to effective epidemic and pandemic prevention. After the ZIKV, the new Brazilian government actively dismantled the public health system, which led to even worse preparedness to the COVID-19 PHEIC.

Politics and framing: Decisions about ZIKV responses were driven by political intentions, which securitized the disease and framed it as "a war on the mosquito." This was favorable in the speed of the response but neglected the pertinent problems in Brazilian society. Where there was a strong political will to firmly respond to ZIKV, the current Brazilian federal government does not acknowledge the seriousness of the COVID-19 pandemic. Both emergencies show that politics are the driving force behind public health decisions and responses. PHEICs should be managed in a technical manner, based on scientific knowledge, without too much political interference.

Vector control and short-term responses: Vector control policies in the response to ZIKV were useful but not sustainable since structural problems, which were the underlying reason why ZIKV could spread explosively, were not considered. Vector control should not only be a response to a crisis and stagnate after; either it should be a main component of the (inter)national agenda, or the underlying problems should be addressed in order to stop the conditions that manifest the spread of the vector.

Structural problems and inequality: In Brazil, most cases of ZIKV were linked to poverty, limited sanitation, and open storage of standing water. Addressing structural problems of poverty and inequality before and during

(continued)

Box 2.1 (continued)

emergency response will be more long-term and sustainable than a crisis-focused short-term response that concentrates on containment of outbreaks. One of the most salient similarities between the PHEICs of ZIKV and COVID-19 is that it is the people living in poor conditions who are most affected.

Gendered approach: Although the ZIKV PHEIC was all about women and babies, the responses and recommendations did not take into account a gendered approach. The responses to the COVID-19 PHEIC also disproportionately burden women. The effects of emergency response policies on women should be considered specifically because it often includes an unrecognized extra load on women's everyday life. Gender planning, gender analysis, and gender thinking should be incorporated in outbreak response.

Research: The international collaboration between researchers following the declaration of the ZIKV PHEIC was very effective. However, the social science research had to be incorporated from the beginning of the response efforts, and treatment and vaccine testing did not receive enough attention since the research evolved after the virus had already died away. There need to be shorter cycles from research into practice, and research should be more actively translated into actual policies to have long-lasting effects. The COVID-19 PHEIC highlights the fact that research into (re-)emerging pathogens in between emergencies could significantly improve emergency preparedness.

Global health architecture: The IHR provided a useful platform to respond to the PHEIC of ZIKV, since it worked as a motor to stimulate research, attention, and funding, yet it also showed the weaknesses of the global health architecture. The COVID-19 PHEIC seems to pose similar challenges as the ZIKV PHEIC, highlighting that several aspects need to be strengthened in the global health architecture, including greater consistency and harmonization of protocols within and between countries, a stronger focus on gender, and core capacities such as surveillance, diagnostics, risk communication, and community engagement.

Communication and Uncertainty in Times of a PHEIC

Declaring the ZIKV crisis, a PHEIC was all about uncertainty, since the declaration was based on what was *not* known about the possible association between the clusters of microcephaly, Guillain–Barré syndrome and other neurological defects and the ZIKV epidemic (ID4, ID5, ID6). The declaration fueled emergency research specifically focused on this uncertainty. At the beginning of the crisis, there was much media attention to the emergency, though the national and global focus differed. On the federal level, the media attention focused on "the war on the

Table 2.1 Overview of research participants

ID number	Organization or function	Description of area(s) of work and experience relevant to the study
ID1	Brazilian Ministry of Health	Surveillance and communicable diseases
ID2	Researcher at Brazilian Research Institution	Epidemiological surveillance
ID3	Researcher at Brazilian University	International relations
ID4	International Brazilian researcher	International relations
ID5	WHO	Global Health Security
ID6	WHO	Emergency Committee
ID7	WHO	Emergency Committee
ID8	International researcher	Politics and international relations
ID9	International researcher	Global health ethics
ID10	International researcher	Global health security, global health governance, infectious disease epidemiology
ID11	International researcher	Epidemiology, disability
ID12	International researcher	Epidemiology and global health, consortia
ID13	PAHO (regional office of WHO)	Public health, finance

mosquito." The Brazilian government tried to reduce uncertainty using response methods focused on vector control that did not require any new knowledge (ID2, ID10). Globally, emotive pictures of women with babies affected with microcephaly dominated the media. Although women and babies were instrumentalized in the global media images, it fueled global attention and research funding related to the ZIKV PHEIC (ID5, ID10). Despite the attention the crisis got in the beginning, the media lost interest over time. Underlying problems of the epidemic and the long-term consequences to the families affected did not receive enough attention, complicating the guarantee of fundamental rights and fulfillment of promises of the affected families (ID1). In the uncertainty and confusion, clinicians and other health workers not always knew well how to communicate the uncertainty to affected families. Therefore, informal support networks and associations that evolved during the PHEIC, such as WhatsApp groups of mothers with affected babies, helped disseminate information among those affected (ID1, ID4, ID11).

> *Social networks allowed families a capacity of articulations which resulted in the creation of associations of mothers and family members who exercised, legitimated and pressured for rights, health and social assistance. The media also had a role in shedding light on the problem. However, the agenda, over time, lost media interest and this fact was identified by families as a problem, as it became more difficult for them to guarantee some basic rights and the fulfillment of some promises when they left the daily debate.* (ID1)

Further problems with uncertainty showed that the initial risk estimates were too high, since the seroprevalence was unknown. It was not communicated clearly that 80% of the people infected were asymptomatic. This resulted in fear and the drastic recommendation to not get pregnant for 2 years, highlighting the need for rational policies based on precise risk estimates rather than fear (ID4, ID5, ID9).

> *... everyone says 'it could do anything' ... everyone is really focused on uncertainty, but it is not as uncertain as people think. One of the big lessons we need to learn is that things are uncertain when the emergency starts, but as I mentioned, it is always almost the case that the worst cases are detected first, so things are usually less risky than they appear. And if we remember that it is not as uncertain as we fear, we can make more rational policies.* (ID9)

Compared to the strong war-language used in the communication during the ZIKV PHEIC which stressed the gravity of the crisis, the Brazilian government's communication in the current COVID-19 pandemic is chaotic and undermines the effects of the pandemic. The government's higher levels give advices contradictive to the recommendations made by (international) public health institutions. The PHEIC of ZIKV was declared about the corresponding uncertainties, and the responses were focused on reducing these uncertainties using scientific knowledge. In contrast, now the contradictive messages increase the tensions concerning the COVID-19 PHEIC. These factors impede attempts to promote and contain the virus (ID1, ID4, ID11).

> *COVID-19 finds Brazil in the midst of a political crisis, with a federal government that has so far defined no policy to confront the epidemic, on the contrary, encourages the opening of trade and services, propagates unproven drug benefits,* etc. ... *There is an incentive to discredit science with systematic attacks on researchers and research and teaching institutions.* (ID1)

Uncertainties play major roles in PHEICs. The ZIKV PHEIC was declared *because of* the uncertainties. During the current COVID-19 pandemic, although not declared *because of* the uncertainties, there are major gaps in scientific knowledge about the disease. This highlights the value and need for a new international, interdisciplinary scientific union in which data is mapped and shared extensively and serves as a new preparedness paradigm (Stuckelberger & Urbina, 2020). Furthermore, communication and the involvement of (new social) media relevant to the communities affected should be strengthened. This can be used more creatively to enhance clear risk communication and cease the circulation of misinformation (Gillespie et al., 2016; Jacobsen et al., 2016). The fact that uncertainties played an essential role in declaring some emergencies as a PHEIC, whereas in others this was not seen as a reason, shows that there is significant inconsistency in the application of the criteria for declaring a PHEIC. This asks for more transparency in the Emergency Committees and guidelines with standardized definitions and implementations of the IHR PHEIC criteria (ID7) (Eccleston-Turner & Kamradt-Scott, 2019).

Politics and Framing of PHEICs

The political context of Brazil in 2016 together with the upcoming Olympic Games in Rio de Janeiro 2016 stimulated the political commitment to understand the gravity of the crisis and mitigate the impacts of the PHEIC. Political factors, therefore, led to accelerated response efforts (ID1, ID2, ID3, ID5, ID10). The Brazilian government framed the ZIKV crisis as "a war on the mosquito" to show that it could effectively handle the emergency and that it was capable of leading the country in times of crisis. Using war-language can be misleading as it draws attention to short-term consequences and responses, thus undermining the underlying structural problems. The securitization framing led to responses that silenced the underlying social determinants which played a significant role in the initial spread of ZIKV. It showed that during a PHEIC, political willingness to respond effectively shapes the response efforts (ID3, ID4, ID10, ID12).

> *During the Zika outbreak, the crisis that Dilma Rousseff was facing, was a really pertinent context to securitizing the disease. We know that securitizing something and creating an enemy which then can be combatted is a really effective fiscal tool for governments ... you can then show how you, as an administration, can overcome it, demonstrating your legitimacy to be able to lead a government ... so, this war narrative was used to improve their political principals.* (ID10)

The initial focus of the ZIKV emergency response was reduced to intensified vector control for the *Aedes aegypti* mosquito. The integrative vector control measures, which included a combination of government, health actors, community, and individual efforts, were effective in killing up to 90% of the mosquitos in Brazil. However, vector control was only a short-term solution since it did not address the conditions which made the vector initially spread (ID1, ID4, ID7, ID9, ID10). Once the crisis ceased, attention and funding faded away, which meant that vector control efforts stagnated, and the vector could spread again (ID1, ID10). Therefore, the government's intense focus on vector control as a public health intervention to stop the spread of ZIKV proves not to be sustainable (ID9, ID10).

> *Vector control policies are useful, but they are not solving the problem, they are putting a plaster on it rather than actually addressing the fact that some people need to store up water because they do not have running water in their house, or inadequate housing, which means that people do not have screens or proper air-condition. There is a tension between the short-term response to Zika and the thinking about the longer term of how to minimize the impact of arboviruses more broadly.* (ID10)

In the ZIKV PHEIC, the Brazilian government notified the emergency early, shared necessary data and translated the Emergency Committee's recommendations well, which led to the fact that politicians mostly let the ZIKV crisis be a technical issue, taking scientific research seriously in their response (ID6). The scientific research considered in the responses primarily focused on clinical research rather than social research about underlying social problems (ID4, ID7). The current president of Brazil is doing precisely the opposite of using war-language and refers to the COVID-19 as "just a little flu" (Ponce, 2020). The current federal government does often not take existing scientific knowledge actively into account and reduces the capacity of the Ministry of Health. Additionally, the Brazilian health system is actively dismantled by the new government since the ZIKV crisis—cutting in capacity, funding, and resources—which complicates an effective response to the COVID-19 pandemic (ID1, ID2, ID3, ID4, ID6, ID11). Measurements to contain the virus and the economy are dichotomously divided, and the virus is not seen as a health crisis but as a threat to the economy. This viewpoint resulted in chaotic management of the COVID-19 PHEIC. Currently, there is no coordinated political response to contain the spread of the virus, the health system is overwhelmed and inequalities are widened (ID1, ID2, ID4, ID7, ID10) (Barberia & Gómez, 2020; Ferigato et al., 2020; Zilla, 2020). The uncoordinated political response and political stance against the public health measures also overturned the individual willingness to follow measures against to spread of COVID-19, resulting in Brazil being one of the epicenters of the pandemic (de Moura et al., 2021).

The sustainability of the lessons learned during the ZIKV PHEIC within the Brazilian government is debatable, since much (social science) research is not transposed to actual policy (ID3, ID4). This results in health authorities having learned from the ZIKV emergency and knowing what to do in future emergencies, but unable to apply these lessons. Their hands are tied because the politicians currently in place are different from the ones during the ZIKV crisis (ID4). On paper, Brazil could have done well in reacting to the COVID-19 pandemic: it had recent scientific and political experiences with responding to a PHEIC, and it has a relatively strong universal health system that serves up to 80% of the population. However, time tells that the health system is now overwhelmed by COVID-19 patients, the government takes contradictive decisions to scientific evidence, and the lessons learned about underlying structural problems are not taken into account in policymaking, resulting in vulnerable groups being disproportionately affected (Farr, 2020).

> *What is happening, is that you have new knowledge and lessons learned by researchers and scientists about how diseases are transmitted, how to fight disease and how to involve social movements and patient care organizations into research, all this knowledge. But the question is, is this transposing to actual policy and attention? ... In terms of what we learned, or what Brazil learned, politicians did not learn anything. Actually, because the politicians who are there now, are very different from the ones who were there during the ZIKV crisis.* (ID4)

For an effective response, public health crises should be managed in a more technical rather than political manner, where decisions are evidence-based and take into account the broader aspects of socio-economic and gender effects (ID6, ID7). Instead of evidence-based decisions, decisions are often based on political ideology, which is not sustainable on the long-term. This stresses the fact that ideological prejudice should not affect the way of dealing with health crises. We should rather listen to experts and people in the field, giving them enough autonomy and resources to do their work. Additionally, there should be space for dialogue with the general public and communities when responses and policies are formulated (ID4, ID6, ID7).

Like public health interventions, PHEIC declarations should be based on science, rather than be politically framed (Mullen et al., 2020). When comparing the PHEIC declarations for the Ebola virus diseases (EVD) in 2014 and the ZIKV in 2016, we see that those declarations are partly based on political framing. The painful lesson learned from the EVD PHEIC was that the declaration and response to the emergency came far too late, which resulted in harsh criticism of the WHO. Contradictorily, in 2016, the WHO declared ZIKV in Brazil and its possible consequences a PHEIC before even knowing the cause of the condition of concern.

ZIKV was securitized with the EVD still fresh in mind by global and local politicians and organizations, and thus shaped by their intention to not make the same mistake twice (Hayden, 2016). Political pressure also exceeds the fact that the WHO is dependent on powerful political donors outside its member states and is thus sensitive to these donors' political interference (Burkle, 2020). Therefore, there is a great need for transparency and consistency in applying the IHR and PHEIC declarations, where guidelines and protocols are uniformly applied and where decisions are made based on science, without much political interference.

Preparedness and Surveillance

The epidemiological surveillance systems in place in Brazil at the time of the ZIKV outbreak rapidly and adequately notified that there was an unusual increase in the cases of microcephaly, which facilitated early organization of the emergency response. Shortly after the notification, investigation of cases was started and partnerships with research institutions like Fiocruz and universities were established (ID1, ID5, ID6). However, the notifications were made on basis of standard measurements that might not have been applicable to the affected population (ID9). The universal public health system in Brazil—Sistema Único da Saúde (SUS) in Portuguese—provided a quality basis for the response to the PHEIC in Brazil through universal access, a strong primary care system and the community health workers structure (ID2, ID3, ID10, ID11). Although the surveillance and public health systems in Brazil enabled an early response to the ZIKV crisis, the country was not prepared for an emergency with the characteristics of ZIKV: the capacity was insufficient outside the big cities, and the overall social determinants of health in Brazil that were the underlying reasons for the spread of the epidemic needed to be improved for a better national response (ID1, ID2, ID3, ID5, ID9).

It is a structural problem in public health crises that very little investment is made in surveillance and preparedness compared to the money spent on the response (ID7, ID9, ID10). Good governance and leadership regarding preparedness is needed to align the policies in place with the economic and technical capacity to respond effectively to a public health emergency (ID7, ID12). In line with this, vaccine trial preparedness and research preparedness are essential to improve the response (ID9). To strengthen the global epidemic and pandemic preparedness, standard preparedness protocols, including vaccine trial protocols, should be available, practiced, and evaluated (ID7, ID9).

> *I think that we have no choice but to strengthen the preparedness aspects of conscious capacities to engage in epidemic and pandemic prevention, control, and response ... all the aspects of disease outbreak response at the preparedness level need to be strengthened and need more investments, as opposed to just looking at them when we have the crisis in our face.* (ID7)

When comparing the preparedness to ZIKV and COVID-19, it has to be acknowledged that they are two very different crises, as the diseases and way of transmission are not comparable. Since Brazil has years of experience in fighting dengue, a vector-borne disease transmitted by the same mosquito as ZIKV, they were more inclined to understand how to respond to the ZIKV PHEIC by increasing vector control. COVID-19 is a new respiratory disease, in which Brazil and many other countries do not have much experience. Therefore, it could be stated that the mental preparedness on how to respond to the ZIKV PHEIC was much greater than to the COVID-19 PHEIC (ID12). Although the experiences with ZIKV offered health workers and politicians experience in PHEICs and should have enabled more mature communication strategies, the political decisions of the current government worsen the preparedness and the capacity of an effective response (ID2, ID5, ID1).

> *My neutrality [to the question if Brazil was better prepared for a next PHEIC after the experience of ZIKV] is due to the fact that theory contradicts reality. In theory, Brazil would be better prepared. In practice, due to the position of the federal government, such fact did not become reality.* (ID1)

To effectively operate, nation states should actively comply with the IHR, strengthening their ability to prevent, prepare, and react to emergencies. Although the WHO member states are obliged to follow the IHR, many countries have poorly implemented its core capacities: a recent study showed that as few as half of 182 countries had strong operational readiness capacities in place (Kandel et al., 2020). In response to this fact, the Global Health Security Agenda (GHSA) was launched in 2014 (Burkle, 2015). The GHSA is an international collaborative effort to support countries to achieve the core capacities of the IHR regulations and aims to adequately prevent, detect, and respond to PHEIC (Global Health Security Agenda, 2021). The effort embodies a broad range of actors, including international organizations, 69 countries, and public and private partners (GHRF Commission, 2016; Wolicki et al., 2016). The GHSA provides a framework that acknowledges the importance of effectively preventing, detecting, and responding to outbreaks, rather than only reporting public health emergencies (Wolicki et al., 2016). Complying more strictly to the IHR, the world could have responded more adequately to the COVID-19 crisis, but instead, the crisis clearly showed a lack of preparedness (Ball, 2020).

> *…there was, or still is, a challenge to what extent the capacities that countries are supposed to have in place to effectively respond, are actually in place. In other words, I do not think that there is an optimum monitoring process … We need greater consistency and harmonization of how protocols actually operate at country level, because there is a lot of unevenness … It will require strong, difficult political negotiations between let's say the WHO and governments. It will not be easy, but I think it is necessary.* (ID7)

Poor implementation of the IHR core capacities is especially the case in resource-poor and vulnerable countries, where there are other national priorities and a lack of recourses to develop preparedness (Kandel et al., 2020; Kluge et al., 2018). This is relevant for the entire globe, as "globally we are only as strong as our weakest link in the chain of surveillance" (Wolicki et al., 2016, p. 187). Ironically, it is primarily countries at a low risk that developed sufficient surveillance capacities. Therefore, a more substantial legal basis that enforces countries to address the gaps in their health and surveillance systems is needed (Kluge et al., 2018). To stimulate enforcement, the global health architecture could use a bottom-up approach in which the civil society is engaged to hold nation states to account in following the IHR (Gostin & Katz, 2016). Enhancing the global preparedness by strengthening the core capacities of the IHR at the national level can only be done when local readiness is improved, requiring a long-term process of change. Kekulé (2015) proposes that epidemic preparedness should be included in international development policies. It is essential to acknowledge the financial costs that come with enhancing preparedness. Reviewing the proportion of financial resources spent on preparedness and crisis response should be promoted. The results highlighted that investing in a prepared and robust health system is more sustainable and cost-effective than rushed emergency mitigations. As the ZIKV PHEIC showed on a small scale, the COVID-19 pandemic clarifies that underfunded, understaffed, and privatized health systems were not prepared to, and capable of handling a PHEIC of this scale (Caduff, 2020). In the end, preparedness in the form of upfront health system investment will mitigate the socio-economic consequences of PHEICs (Kluge et al., 2018).

Our study highlighted that next to the promotion of international policies that focus on preparedness, it is crucial to recognize that countries have different approaches in controlling outbreaks. The global network that enables quick notification of infectious diseases should be enhanced, using solid standardized protocols consistently lived up to, monitored, and evaluated (Kluge et al., 2018). To stimulate this enhancement, there is a need for more (binding) international treaties, and strengthening of the authority of the WHO (Ball, 2020). Context matters. This is, for example, seen in the different effectiveness rates of the recent lockdowns that were declared to prevent the spread of COVID-19. What works in one country may not be suitable in another country (Caduff, 2020; Mendenhall, 2020; Stott, 2020). Enhancing preparedness in individual countries also requires strong political will of national governments. This study highlights that governments' ideologies and political motivations are for a great deal shaping the emergency preparedness and public health interventions in a country, as discussed in section "Communication and Uncertainty in Times of a PHEIC". Thus, the key to a strong global preparedness and surveillance system has robust protocols that can be slightly adapted to the context, to ensure consistency and to recognize that context matters.

International Research Collaboration

The declaration of the possible association between ZIKV and clusters of microcephaly and Guillain–Barré syndrome as a PHEIC triggered effective global collaboration, networking, and data sharing in which countries were working together to rapidly understand the link between ZIKV infection and microcephaly and other neurological effects (ID2, ID3, ID4, ID5, ID6, ID8, ID11, ID12, ID13). The declaration of ZIKV as a PHEIC attracted attention and funding for collaboration between international and Brazilian research institutes, and additionally, three EU-funded ZIKV consortia were formed. Although the global collaboration proved to be adequate, its challenges shed light on the importance of including local communities and sharing study results with research participants. It also highlighted that "parachuting researchers"—those who come at the point of the crisis to extract knowledge but do not show the benefits of the research to participants and the local population—should be avoided (ID1, ID4, ID10, ID11, ID12): research participation should be participatory and ethically conscious, with clear communicated benefits for the population (ID4, ID9). The ZIKV PHEIC showed that it is crucial to analyze social data next to clinical, epidemiological, and surveillance data during public health emergencies. During the ZIKV PHEIC, the realization of the importance of social data that addressed structural problems came gradually. In contrast, responses could have been more effective and sustainable if they were actively considered from the beginning (ID7).

> *We need to have a better understanding of people's perceptions and people's practices, in terms of the relevance to infectious diseases ... when we have a crisis and we then try to collect data, you miss a lot of the history of where this data might come from, which is extremely important. In terms of improving systems I think there needs to be a much stronger focus on how we build data systems that focus on social aspects of disease outbreaks and pandemics, because we struggle tremendously early on in these responses to see what we know and what we can draw on.* (ID7)

The record speed on which international scientific research was generated resulted from the attention, funding, and resources stimulated by the global recognition of the emergency (Larrandaburu et al., 2017). However, public interest and funding faded away after the immediate emergency, and treatment and vaccine testing were not moved into action quickly since the virus died away (ID9, ID11). The comparison between the ZIKV and COVID-19 PHEIC, in which scientific research was used in a completely different manner by governments, shows the importance of short cycles between research and policymakers (ID3, ID4, ID11). This shows the persistent flaws of the global health architecture: there are attention and funding in times of crisis, but although ZIKV was discovered more than 70 years ago and there have been several outbreaks, there is still no vaccine or treatment, and the long-term consequences of the emergency are neglected (Hayden, 2016; Jamrozik & Selgelid, 2018; Smith & Silva, 2015). Short cycles between researchers and policymakers ensure that research is translated into policies and influences and prioritizes the political agenda. During COVID-19, international research collaboration evolved quickly after the emergency started (ID12). But again, research preparedness was far to be sought. Although there have been severe outbreaks with other coronaviruses like SARS and MERS, there is limited public health research for coronaviruses. This highlights the importance of researching in between emergencies, preparing for the next emergency (ID9). International research preparedness, including ethical preparedness, is also a central point that needs to be improved in the global health architecture.

Structural Problems and Inequality

Brazil copes with structural problems concerning poverty and inequality, sexual and reproductive rights, poor sanitation, waste management and infrastructure. These long-term issues facilitated the fast rate of infection and transmission of ZIKV (ID1–ID13). For example, in Recife, a city in Northeastern Brazil, most cases were concentrated in poor living conditions. This is in line with the conception that children affected by the consequences of ZIKV are most likely to be born in low socio-economic households (ID1, ID5, ID7, ID9, ID10, ID11). These families, therefore, face "just another" burden and are unequally economically affected (ID4, ID11).

Since the national and to a great extent also the international responses were focused on vector control, important long-term issues were initially glossed over. Therefore, the responses did not result in effective structural change in Brazilian society (ID4, ID7, ID10). It could be stated that the focus on vector control and the attention to structural problems were not in balance in the emergency response (ID9). To respond with long-term solutions, governments should consider the structural issues that communities face and facilitate adequate emergency response to an infectious disease outbreak (ID3). In line with that, public health crises can turn into socio-economic crises very quickly. This needs to be recognized and integrated very early on in the crisis response to maintain effective public health interventions (ID7). PHEICs do not only harm the health of people, but they also pose significant threats to economic and social stability. When with ZIKV, the socio-economic risks mainly played in the background and came gradually to the surface, the public health measurements to contain the spread of COVID-19 disrupt economic and socially valuable activities immediately in noticeable ways (Bloom & Cadarette, 2019).

> *Every time this [an infectious disease outbreak] happens, what we see is that inequality made manifest. It is not the infection that is killing people, it is inequality and poverty.* (ID9)
>
> *Local populations learnt about the need to treat standing water and cover wherever possible. However, it is unlikely that this is generally sustained, as the government undertook some of the treatment measures and mosquito eradication measures that the local population would not be able to afford.* (ID5)

The structural issues that played a major role in the spread of ZIKV and resulted in disproportionately affected groups are now becoming problematic again during the COVID-19 PHEIC. This shows that structural change did not happen after the ZIKV PHEIC. The same groups that were affected most by ZIKV are the ones most at risk for COVID-19 as well: the poorest and most deprived and the ones without proper housing and sanitation (ID4, ID9, ID10, ID11).

> *Children affected are much more likely to be born in low socio-economic households, and that has made it much more difficult for the families to cope. ... A lot of the women we interviewed, having a severely disabled child was now just one of the issues they were facing in their lives ... it is important to understand that ZIKV was disproportionately affecting poor people who were already having it difficult. And that is probably going to be true with COVID-19 as well; it will widen inequalities.* (ID11)

The key lessons presented in our study accentuate the imbalance between short-term emergency responses and sustainable long-term responses. In the ZIKV PHEIC, one main underlying problem was Brazil's inequality: the highest infection rates were found among black and brown women of low socio-economic status, living in poor and densely populated areas or desolated backlands (Diniz et al., 2016). Currently, social, racial, and gender inequalities are again manifesting the spread of disease, making Brazil one of the epicenters of the COVID-19 pandemic. As an example: dying of COVID-19 is 62% more likely for Blacks in Sao Paolo than Whites (Barber, 2020). But anew, the interventions focus on individual behavior, neglecting structural issues of inequality (Reis-Castro & Nogueira, 2020). A great part of the Brazilian population lives in jam-packed urban areas, with poor access to clean water and sanitation, making it difficult to practice social distancing or follow hygiene recommendations. A SARS-CoV-2 antibody prevalence study in Brazil confirmed that prevalence was unevenly distributed per region and was highest in the poorest areas. The prevalence proved to be strongly associated with Indigenous ancestry and low socio-economic status (Hallal et al., 2020). Inequality is not only a driving force in the spread of infectious diseases but also deepened by the consequences of outbreaks. There is an urgent need to acknowledge this in response to efforts and policies to protect those that are already vulnerable and burdened by everyday challenges. A recent study on the (mis-)managing of pandemics showed that governments that emphasize the importance of public health instead of focusing on short-term economic consequences obtained a higher approval over time (Herrera et al., 2020). Governments must maintain a good balance in focus on improving public health, addressing structural (underlying) problems, and acknowledging the socio-economic consequences of a PHEIC.

Understanding the history and context of the populations affected by an outbreak is fundamental when formulating effective public health measures; our study aims to contribute to that. To achieve this, there should be a better balance in focus on the epidemiological data and the long-term social and economic effects within the IHR, the Emergency Committees' recommendations, and national governments. More funding and attention to social science research before and during epidemics are needed. The inclusion of social sciences in outbreak preparedness and management should also be represented on a global level, including more social scientists in the WHO would therefore be a great start to set the example (Kekulé, 2015; Passos et al., 2020).

A Gendered Approach

The focus on vector control during the ZIKV PHEIC did not take into consideration the structural problems that the Brazilian society faces, including the lack of sexual and reproductive rights. The association between microcephaly and ZIKV made women of reproductive age the most vulnerable group in the ZIKV outbreak, resulting in the advice to not get pregnant for 2 years to avoid the risk of giving birth to a baby suffering from CZS. When viewed from a gendered approach, more effective recommendations would include better access to antenatal care for women in low-resource settings and an overall broad choice of reproductive options (ID9, ID10, ID11).

Furthermore, the response efforts did not recognize that the recommendations and interventions included heavily gendered activities. Both the vector control activities and the contraception decision generally fall onto women. In most cases, it is the woman who has more domestic responsibilities and thus bears the extra load of keeping the house free from mosquitos and improving the water and sanitation situation. Women of reproductive age and pregnant women were most vulnerable during the ZIKV outbreak. Yet, they were not included in the decision-making process of formulating responses, and the impacts of vector control policies on them were largely neglected. This highlights the importance of having a gendered approach when public health policies and emergency responses are formulated (ID10). Recently, a study was published about the role of gender in Zika prevention behaviors in the Dominican Republic and their results stressed that understanding the gendered roles in prevention is needed to strengthen prevention and control measures. To integrate gender in prevention and control programs, taking the local context into account, they suggested to tailor activities for men, women, and couples. Hereby it is important to not exploit local existing gender roles (Gurman et al., 2020).

> *During the ZIKV outbreak, it was all about women. It was all about protecting women from having babies with microcephaly. So, on paper, it was all about women, but actually it was not about women at all. The government of Brazil did nothing to try and incorporate gender planning, gender analysis and gender thinking into how they responded to the outbreak.* (ID10)

In the current COVID-19 pandemic, we see once again that women are disproportionately burdened with the response measures taken; it is mostly them, following the gendered norms, who have to manage the extra childcare, the house chores that are the result of lockdown measurements, and the community work. However, this is not acknowledged and recognized enough, since there is no extra support for women and no difference in how women are expected to continue working in informal jobs (ID10).

Governments should prioritize the embodiment of gender analysis in preparedness and response efforts to ensure that recommendations and interventions are sustainable and promote equity in gender and health (Wenham et al., 2020). Smith showed in a case study that during the EVD outbreak in 2014, mainstreaming gender in response efforts, engaging women in the policy decision-making processes of a local NGO, and putting them at the center of the response were effective ways of including a gendered approach in emergency responses. She also highlighted that including gender in preparedness policies is essential and in line with an enhanced focus on the structural problems and socio-economic consequences that play a role in PHEICs (Smith, 2019). These are essential lessons from the EVD PHEIC. It is concerning that they are not effectively applied in the responses to the ZIKV PHEIC and the COVID-19 PHEIC, where structural gender inequalities are still left out of the crisis response, revealing the "conspicuous invisibility of women" in the global health architecture (Davies & Bennett, 2016; Wenham et al., 2020). The ZIKV and COVID-19 PHEICs show the disproportional burden women can face from both the infection and the prevention and control measures. This underlines the rationale of including a gendered approach more actively in the global health architecture, especially in the IHR. This will stimulate the recognition of gendered dimensions in national policies and local initiatives (Smith, 2019). Both a bottom-up and top-down approach on the inclusion of a gendered approach is therefore needed.

ZIKV and the COVID-19 Pandemic: A Reflection to the Key Concepts of the Book

The comparison between the ZIKV PHEIC and the COVID-19 pandemic in this chapter shows how important a solid global health architecture is for disease outbreak preparedness and response. Although countries must comply to the IHR and effective risk communication is one of its core capacities, this research showed that in the end, the effectiveness highly depends on the political will of the national leaders in place. The pillars set by the WHO for epidemic and pandemic response are not easily and quickly translated to national level, often resulting in an uneven performance of the pillars. Besides good governance and leadership and political will, it is also needed that the community trusts government authorities. In line with the results of our study, governments are more trusted when they maintain a good balance between the focus on public health and the underlying socio-economic causes and consequences. Thus, the key concept of "trust" is highlighted in this chapter by showing the importance of political will of governments to adequately respond to PHEICs and the importance of clear evidence-based policies to induce effective individual and community behavior change.

As the paragraph above highlights, there should be more consistency between all pillars of epidemic response at country level. This requires clear and consistent protocols that are monitored and evaluated. Forcing countries to follow the IHR can only be reached through good governance and leadership, political will, and international negotiations. In the current COVID-19 PHEIC, although the interventions recommended are very different than in the ZIKV PHEIC, similar challenges within the functioning of the global health architecture are seen: there is a great variety in countries' capacities to translate the recommendations by the WHO, great differences in the application of principles and protocols and challenges with coordination at country level. However, as highlighted in section "Politics and Framing of PHEICs", context matters. Therefore, the WHO could stimulate social science research to make the IHR better work in a variety of contexts and cultures.

As the PHEICs in this chapter clearly showed, social and behavioral determinants both affect and are affected by public health emergencies. The ZIKV PHEIC was partially fueled by the socio-economic inequalities in Brazil, and the COVID-19 pandemic is widening these inequalities even more. The results of our research highlighted that the inclusion of social science in emergency preparedness and response is needed to understand how underlying problems play a role in the emergency. When these problems are acknowledged early on in the emergency, and the history and context of the populations affected are understood, more effective policies could be formulated. As the ZIKV PHEIC showed, it was in the end not effective to only focus on vector control measures that individuals and communities themselves could not maintain after the emergency attention of the government faded away. Since control and prevention of most infectious diseases rely on behavior change on individual level, policymakers should rather engage the community to find solutions to underlying problems to prevent new emergencies. Our research highlighted the importance of taking into account not only the variety of different cultures and contexts but also acknowledging the underlying problems they face. This relates back to the key concepts of "complexity" and "culture" in this book.

Our research also showed the importance of a gendered approach during emergency preparedness and response measures. The ZIKV PHEIC perfectly illustrated this, since this epidemic was all about women, but women were not actively engaged in the policymaking processes. We hope that in the near future, women's rights are more actively considered in the global health architecture to ensure that this dripples down in national policies. The concept of "human rights" of this book is therefore reflected in the rationale to more actively include a gendered approach and focus on women's rights in the IHR as well as in national response measures.

The concept of "misinformation and rumors" is reflected in how the Brazilian government used very different approaches to risk communication during the ZIKV PHEIC and the COVID-19 pandemic. The strong focus on "the war on the mosquito" and the policies for the control of ZIKV were mainly based on scientific (but non-social science) research. However, social networks also played a role in sharing information about topics where people felt government and public health information was lacking or not supporting. This fueled misconceptions and rumors. During the COVID-19 pandemic, the current government in Brazil does not make evidence-based decisions, which fuels the spread of rumors, disinformation, and misinformation even more. Not only Brazil, but the world will soon encounter the risks, including new virus variants, that this approach brings.

Conclusion

Our study evaluated the lessons learned of the ZIKV PHEIC and compared and contrasted those to the COVID-19 PHEIC in Brazil based on experiences, opinions, and experts' recommendations in the field. The ZIKV and COVID-19 PHEIC therefore served as case studies that facilitated the opportunity to learn from a passed PHEIC and compare it to a current PHEIC. One of the main lessons from both cases is that governments should step away from strong ideologies in times of a PHEIC, to ensure an evidence-based response rather than a politically shaped response. The focus on how structural problems regarding socio-economic status and poverty play a role in PHEICs should be enhanced to formulate sustainable emergency responses. By all means, including a gendered approach to national policies and into the global health architecture is needed to recognize that women are often disproportionally burdened by risks of diseases and emergency measures taken. All of these aspects are important to consider when we want to strengthen the response of the global health architecture to epidemics and pandemics. Just as importantly, we should recognize that investing in preparedness will, in the long-term, be more effective and more economic.

References

de Araújo, T. V. B., Rodrigues, L. C., de Alencar Ximenes, R. A., de Barros Miranda-Filho, D., Montarroyos, U. R., de Melo, A. P. L., Valongueiro, S., de Albuquerque, M. F. P. M., Souza, W. V., Braga, C., Filho, S. P. B., Cordeiro, M. T., Vazquez, E., Di Cavalcanti Souza Cruz, D., Henriques, C. M. P., Bezerra, L. C. A., da Silva Castanha, P. M., Dhalia, R., Marques-Júnior, E. T. A., & Martelli, C. M. T. (2016). Association between Zika virus infection and microcephaly in Brazil, January to May, 2016: Preliminary report of a case-control study. *The Lancet Infectious Diseases, 16*(12), 1356–1363. https://doi.org/10.1016/S1473-3099(16)30318-8

Avelino-Silva, V. I., & Kallas, E. G. (2018). Untold stories of the Zika virus epidemic in Brazil. *Reviews in Medical Virology, 28*(6), 1–9. https://doi.org/10.1002/rmv.2000

Ball, P. (2020). Pandemic science and politics. *The Lancet, 396*(10246), 229–230. https://doi.org/10.1016/s0140-6736(20)31594-4

Barber, S. (2020). Death by racism. *The Lancet Infectious Diseases, 20*(8), 903. https://doi.org/10.1016/S1473-3099(20)30567-3

Barberia, L. G., & Gómez, E. J. (2020). Political and institutional perils of Brazil's COVID-19 crisis. *The Lancet, 396*(10248), 367–368. https://doi.org/10.1016/S0140-6736(20)31681-0

Bedford, J., Enria, D., Giesecke, J., Heymann, D. L., Ihekweazu, C., Kobinger, G., Lane, H. C., Memish, Z., Oh, M., don Sall, A. A., Schuchat, A., Ungchusak, K., & Wieler, L. H. (2020). COVID-19: Towards controlling of a pandemic. *The Lancet, 395*(10229), 1015–1018. https://doi.org/10.1016/S0140-6736(20)30673-5

Bloom, D. E., & Cadarette, D. (2019). Infectious disease threats in the twenty-first century: Strengthening the global response. *Frontiers in Immunology, 10*, 549. https://doi.org/10.3389/fimmu.2019.00549

Brady, O. J., Osgood-Zimmerman, A., Kassebaum, N. J., Ray, S. E., De Araùjo, V. E. M., Da Nóbrega, A. A., Frutuoso, L. C. V., Lecca, R. C. R., Stevens, A., De Oliveira, B. Z., De Lima, J. M., Bogoch, I. I., Mayaud, P., Jaenisch, T., Mokdad, A. H., Murray, C. J. L., Hay, S. I., Reiner, R. C., & Marinho, F. (2019). The association between Zika virus infection and microcephaly in Brazil 2015–2017: An observational analysis of over 4 million births. *PLoS Medicine, 16*(3), 1–21. https://doi.org/10.1371/journal.pmed.1002755

Brasil, P., Pereira, J. P., Moreira, M. E., Nogueira, R. M. R., Damasceno, L., Wakimoto, M., Rabello, R. S., Valderramos, S. G., Halai, U. A., Salles, T. S., Zin, A. A., Horovitz, D., Daltro, P., Boechat, M., Gabaglia, C. R., De Sequeira, P. C., Pilotto, J. H., Medialdea-Carrera, R., Da Cunha, D. C., … Nielsen-Saines, K. (2016). Zika virus infection in pregnant women in Rio de Janeiro. *New England Journal of Medicine, 375*(24), 2321–2334. https://doi.org/10.1056/NEJMoa1602412

Bueno, F. T. C. (2017). Health surveillance and response on a regional scale: A preliminary study of the Zika virus fever case. *Ciencia e Saude Coletiva, 22*(7), 2305–2314. https://doi.org/10.1590/1413-81232017227.07012017

Burkle, F. M. (2015). Global health security demands a strong International Health Regulations treaty and leadership from a highly resourced World Health Organization. *Disaster Medicine and Public Health Preparedness, 9*(5), 568–580. https://doi.org/10.1017/dmp.2015.26

Burkle, F. M. (2020). Political intrusions into the International Health Regulations treaty and its impact on management of rapidly emerging zoonotic pandemics: What history tells us. *Prehospital and Disaster Medicine, 35*(4), 426–430. https://doi.org/10.1017/S1049023X20000515

Caduff, C. (2020). What went wrong: Corona and the world after the full stop. *Medical Anthropology Quarterly, 34*(4), 467–487. https://doi.org/10.1111/maq.12599

Chang, C., Ortiz, K., Ansari, A., & Gershwin, M. E. (2016). The Zika outbreak of the 21st century. *Journal of Autoimmunity, 68*, 1–13. https://doi.org/10.1016/j.jaut.2016.02.006

Davies, S. E., & Bennett, B. (2016). A gendered human rights analysis of Ebola and Zika: Locating gender in global health emergencies. *International Affairs, 92*(5), 1041–1060. https://doi.org/10.1111/1468-2346.12704

Diniz, D., Gumieri, S., Bevilacqua, B. G., Cook, R. J., & Dickens, B. M. (2016). Zika virus infection in Brazil and human rights obligations. *International Journal of Gynecology and Obstetrics, 136*(1), 105–110. https://doi.org/10.1002/ijgo.12018

Eccleston-Turner, M., & Kamradt-Scott, A. (2019). Transparency in IHR emergency committee decision making: The case for reform. *BMJ Global Health, 4*(2), 10–12. https://doi.org/10.1136/bmjgh-2019-001618

Epelboin, S., Dulioust, E., Epelboin, L., Benachi, A., Merlet, F., & Patrat, C. (2017). Zika virus and reproduction: Facts, questions and current management. *Human Reproduction Update, 23*(6), 629–645. https://doi.org/10.1093/humupd/dmx024

Farr, C. (2020). Brazil turned the coronavirus into a political football, with devastating results. *CNBC*. Retrieved from https://www.cnbc.com/2020/07/22/brazil-politics-mixed-messages-hurt-response.html

Ferigato, S., Fernandez, M., Amorim, M., Ambrogi, I., Fernandes, L. M. M., & Pacheco, R. (2020). The Brazilian Government's mistakes in responding to the COVID-19 pandemic. *The Lancet, 396*(10263), 1636. https://doi.org/10.1016/S0140-6736(20)32164-4

Fidler, D. P. (2005). From international sanitary conventions to global health security: The new International Health Regulations. *Chinese Journal of International Law, 4*(2), 325–392. https://doi.org/10.1093/chinesejil/jmi029

Fidler, D. P., & Gostin, L. O. (2006). The new International Health Regulations: An historic development for international law and public health. *Journal of Law, Medicine and Ethics, 34*(1), 85–94. https://doi.org/10.1111/j.1748-720X.2006.00011.x

Fischer, J., & Katz, R. (2010). The revised international health response, A framework for global pandemic. *Global Health Governance, 3*(2), 1–18. https://doi.org/10.1186/1746-1596-9-138

Fraser, B., & Alves, L. (2019). Living with the consequences of Zika virus disease. *The Lancet Child and Adolescent Health, 3*(4), 215–216. https://doi.org/10.1016/S2352-4642(19)30066-5

GHRF Commission (Commission on a Global Health Risk Framework for the Future). (2016). *The neglected dimension of global security: A framework to counter infectious disease crises*. National Academies Press. https://doi.org/10.17226/21891

Giesecke, J., & STAG-IH. (2019). The truth about PHEICs. *Lancet (London, England), S0140-6736(19)31566-1*. https://doi.org/10.1016/S0140-6736(19)31566-1

Gillespie, A., Obregon, R., El Asawi, R., Richey, C., Manoncourt, E., Joshi, K., Naqvi, S., Pouye, A., Safi, N., Chitnis, K., & Quereshi, S. (2016). Social mobilization and community engagement central to the Ebola response in West Africa: Lessons for future public health emergencies. *Global Health Science and Practice, 4*(4), 626–646. https://doi.org/10.9745/GHSP-D-16-00226

Global Health Security Agenda. (2021). *Global Health Security Agenda*. Retrieved from https://ghsagenda.org/

Gostin, L. O., & Katz, R. (2016). The International Health Regulations: The governing framework for global health security. *Milbank Quarterly, 94*(2), 264–313. https://doi.org/10.1111/1468-0009.12186

Gurman, T., Sara, A. B., Lorenzo, F. V., Luis, D., Hunter, G., Maloney, S., Fujita-Conrads, R., & Leontsini, E. (2020). The role of gender in Zika prevention behaviors in the Dominican Republic: Findings and programmatic implications from a qualitative study. *PLoS Neglected Tropical Diseases, 14*(3), 1–17. https://doi.org/10.1371/journal.pntd.0007994

Hallal, P. C., Hartwig, F. P., Horta, B. L., Silveira, M. F., Struchiner, C. J., Vidaletti, L. P., Neumann, N. A., Pellanda, L. C., Dellagostin, O. A., Burattini, M. N., Victora, G. D., Menezes, A. M. B., Barros, F. C., Barros, A. J. D., & Victora, C. G. (2020). SARS-CoV-2 antibody prevalence in Brazil: Results from two successive nationwide serological household surveys. *The Lancet Global Health, 8*(11), e1390–e1398. https://doi.org/10.1016/S2214-109X(20)30387-9

Hayden, E. C. (2016). Spectre of Ebola haunts Zika response. *Nature, 531*(7592), 19. https://doi.org/10.1038/531019a

Herrera, H., Konradt, M., Ordoñez, G., & Trebesch, C. (2020). *Corona politics: The cost of mismanaging pandemics* (Kiel Working Paper, 2165). Retrieved from http://hdl.handle.net/10419/224062

Heymann, D. L., Hodgson, A., Sall, A. A., Freedman, D. O., Staples, J. E., Althabe, F., Baruah, K., Mahmud, G., Kandun, N., Vasconcelos, P. F. C., Bino, S., & Menon, K. U. (2016). Zika virus and microcephaly: Why is this situation a PHEIC? *The Lancet, 387*(10020), 719–721. https://doi.org/10.1016/S0140-6736(16)00320-2

Howard-Jones, N. (1975). *The scientific background of the International Sanitary Conferences, 1851–1938*. World Health Organization.

Jacobsen, K. H., Alonso Aguirre, A., Bailey, C. L., Baranova, A. V., Crooks, A. T., Croitoru, A., Delamater, P. L., Gupta, J., Kehn-Hall, K., Narayanan, A., Pierobon, M., Rowan, K. E., Reid Schwebach, J., Seshaiyer, P., Sklarew, D. M., Stefanidis, A., & Agouris, P. (2016). Lessons from the ebola outbreak: Action items for emerging infectious disease preparedness and response. *EcoHealth, 13*(1), 200–212. https://doi.org/10.1007/s10393-016-1100-5

Jamrozik, E., & Selgelid, M. J. (2018). Ethics, health policy, and Zika: From emergency to global epidemic? *Journal of Medical Ethics, 44*(5), 343–348. https://doi.org/10.1136/medethics-2017-104,389

John Hopkins University (JHU). (2021). *COVID-19 Dashboard by the Center for Systems Science and Engineering (CSSE) at John Hopkins University (JHU)*. Retrieved June 5, 2021, from https://coronavirus.jhu.edu/map.html

Kandel, N., Chungong, S., Omaar, A., & Xing, J. (2020). Health security capacities in the context of COVID-19 outbreak: An analysis of International Health Regulations annual report data from 182 countries. *The Lancet, 395*(10229), 1047–1053. https://doi.org/10.1016/S0140-6736(20)30553-5

Kekulé, A. S. (2015). Learning from ebola virus: How to prevent future epidemics. *Viruses, 7*(7), 3789–3797. https://doi.org/10.3390/v7072797

Kluge, H., Martín-Moreno, J. M., Emiroglu, N., Rodier, G., Kelley, E., Vujnovic, M., & Permanand, G. (2018). Strengthening global health security by embedding the International Health Regulations requirements into national health systems. *BMJ Global Health, 3*(Suppl 1), e000656. https://doi.org/10.1136/bmjgh-2017-000656

Kuper, H., Lyra, T. M., Moreira, M. E. L., Do De Albuquerque, M. S. V., De Araújo, T. V. B., Fernandes, S., Jofre-Bonet, M., Larson, H., De Melo, A. P. L., Mendes, C. H. F., Moreira, M. C. N., Do Nascimento, M. A. F., Penn-Kekana, L., Pimentel, C., Pinto, M., Simas, C., & Valongueiro, S. (2019). Social and economic impacts of congenital ZIKA syndrome in Brazil: Study protocol and rationale for a mixed-methods study [version 2; peer review: 2 approved]. *Wellcome Open Research, 3*, 1–15. https://doi.org/10.12688/wellcomeopenres.14838.1

Larrandaburu, M., Vianna, F. S., Anjos-daSilva, A., Sanseverino, M. T., & Schuler-Faccini, L. (2017). Zika virus infection and congenital anomalies in the Americas: Opportunities for regional action. *Revista Panamericana de Salud Pública, 41*, e174. https://doi.org/10.26633/rpsp.2017.174

van der Linden, V., Pessoa, A., Dobyns, W., James Barkovich, A., van der Linden, H., Rolim Filho, E. L., Ribeiro, E. M., De Carvalho Leal, M., De Araújo Coimbra, P. P., De Fátima Viana Vasco Aragão, M., Verçosa, I., Ventura, C., Ramos, R. C., Sousa Cruz, D. D. C., Cordeiro, M. T., Ribeiro Mota, V. M., Dott, M., Hillard, C., & Moore, C. A. (2016). Description of 13 infants born during October 2015—January 2016 with congenital Zika virus infection without microcephaly at birth—Brazil. *Morbidity and Mortality Weekly Report, 65*(47), 1343–1348. https://doi.org/10.15585/mmwr.mm6547e2

Lowe, R., Barcellos, C., Brasil, P., Cruz, O. G., Honório, N. A., Kuper, H., & Carvalho, M. S. (2018). The Zika virus epidemic in Brazil: From discovery to future implications. *International Journal of Environmental Research and Public Health, 15*(1), 96. https://doi.org/10.3390/ijerph15010096

Mendenhall, E. (2020). The COVID-19 syndemic is not global: Context matters. *The Lancet, 396*(10264), 1731. https://doi.org/10.1016/S0140-6736(20)32218-2

Merianos, A., & Peiris, M. (2005). International Health Regulations (2005). *The Lancet, 366*(9493), 1249–1251. https://doi.org/10.1016/s0140-6736(05)67508-3

Ministério da Saúde - Secretaria de Vigilância em Saúde. (2019). Síndrome congênita associada à infeccção pelo vírus Zika. *Boletim Epidemiológico, Número Esp* (Nov. 2019), 1–30. Retrieved from http://portalarquivos2.saude.gov.br/images/pdf/2019/dezembro/05/be-sindrome-congenita-vfinal.pdf

de Moura, F., Villela, E., López, R. V. M., Sato, A. P. S., de Oliveira, F. M., Waldman, E. A., Van den Bergh, R., Siewe Fodjo, J. N., & Colebunders, R. (2021). COVID-19 outbreak in Brazil: Adherence to national preventive measures and impact on people's lives, an online survey. *BMC Public Health, 21*(1), 1–10. https://doi.org/10.1186/s12889-021-10,222-z

Mullen, L., Potter, C., Gostin, L. O., Cicero, A., & Nuzzo, J. B. (2020). An analysis of International Health Regulations Emergency Committees and Public Health Emergency of International Concern Designations. *BMJ Global Health, 5*(6), e002502. https://doi.org/10.1136/bmjgh-2020-002502

Musso, D., Roche, C., Robin, E., Nhan, T., Teissier, A., & Cao-Lormeau, V.-M. (2015). Potential sexual transmission of Zika virus. *Emerging Infectious Diseases, 21*(2), 359–361. https://doi.org/10.3201/eid2102.141363

Nuttall, I., & Odugleh-Kolev, A. (2012). *International Health Regulations implementation: Ensuring effective responses to public health emergencies: strengthening risk communication capacities of national systems.* World Health Organization (WHO). Retrieved from https://www.who.int/ihr/about/07_risk_communication.pdf

Oliveira, W. K., Carmo, E. H., Henriques, C. M., Coelho, G., Vazques, E., Cortez-Escalante, J., Molina, J., Aldighieri, S., Espinal, M. A., & Dye, C. (2017). Zika virus infection and associated neurologic disorders in Brazil. *New England Journal of Medicine, 376*(16), 1591–1593. https://doi.org/10.1056/NEJMc1608612

Passos, M. J., Matta, G., Lyra, T. M., Moreira, M. E. L., Kuper, H., Penn-Kekana, L., & Mendonça, M. (2020). The promise and pitfalls of social science research in an emergency: Lessons from studying the Zika epidemic in Brazil, 2015–2016. *BMJ Global Health, 5*(4), e002307. https://doi.org/10.1136/bmjgh-2020-002307

Ponce, D. (2020). The impact of coronavirus in Brazil: Politics and the pandemic. *Nature Reviews Nephrology, 16*(9), 483. https://doi.org/10.1038/s41581-020-0327-0

Possas, C. (2016). Zika: What we do and do not know based on the experiences of Brazil. *Epidemiology and Health, 38*(May), e2016023. https://doi.org/10.4178/epih.e2016023

Reis-Castro, L., & Nogueira, C. (2020, April 6). Who should be concerned? Zika as an epidemic about mosquitoes and women (and some reflections on COVID-19). *Somatosphere* (pp. 1–22). Retrieved from http://somatosphere.net/2020/zika-epidemic-mosquitos-women.html/%0AWho

Smith, J. (2019). Overcoming the 'tyranny of the urgent': Integrating gender into disease outbreak preparedness and response. *Gender and Development, 27*(2), 355–369. https://doi.org/10.1080/13552074.2019.1615288

Smith, M. J., & Silva, D. S. (2015). Ethics for pandemics beyond influenza: Ebola, drug-resistant tuberculosis, and anticipating future ethical challenges in pandemic preparedness and response. *Monash Bioethics Review, 33*, 130–147. https://doi.org/10.1007/s40592-015-0038-7

Stott, M. (2020). Pandemic politics: The rebound of Latin America's populists. *Financial Times*. Retrieved from https://www.ft.com/content/3c24bf86-2c47-4939-9477-cefd655d4d48

Stuckelberger, A., & Urbina, M. (2020). WHO International Health Regulations (IHR) vs COVID-19 uncertainty. *Acta Biomedica, 91*(2), 113–117. https://doi.org/10.23750/abm.v91i2.9626

Wenham, C., Smith, J., & Morgan, R. (2020). COVID-19: The gendered impacts of the outbreak. *The Lancet, 395*(10227), 846–848. https://doi.org/10.1016/S0140-6736(20)30526-2

Wolicki, S. B., Nuzzo, J. B., Blazes, D. L., Pitts, D. L., Iskander, J. K., & Tappero, J. W. (2016). Public health surveillance: At the core of the global health security agenda. *Health Security, 14*(3), 185–188. https://doi.org/10.1089/hs.2016.0002

World Health Organization (WHO). (2016a). *International Health Regulations (2005)—Third edition*. World Health Organization.

World Health Organization (WHO). (2016b). *Fifth meeting of the Emergency Committee under the International Health Regulations (2005) regarding microcephaly, other neurological disorders and Zika virus*. Retrieved from https://www.who.int/en/news-room/detail/18-11-2016-fifth-meeting-of-the-emergency-committee-under-the-international-health-regulations-(2005)-regarding-microcephaly-other-neurological-disorders-and-zika-virus

World Health Organization (WHO). (2020a). *Statement on the second meeting of the International Health Regulations (2005) Emergency Committee regarding the outbreak of novel coronavirus (2019-nCoV)*. Retrieved from https://www.who.int/news-room/detail/30-01-2020-statement-on-the-second-meeting-of-the-international-health-regulations-(2005)-emergency-committee-regarding-the-outbreak-of-novel-coronavirus-(2019-ncov)

World Health Organization (WHO). (2020b). *WHO/Europe | Coronavirus disease (COVID-19) outbreak—2019-nCoVoutbreakisanemergencyofinternationalconcern.2005*,2019–2020.Retrieved from http://www.euro.who.int/en/health-topics/health-emergencies/coronavirus-covid-19/news/news/2020/01/2019-ncov-outbreak-is-an-emergency-of-international-concern

World Health Organization (WHO). (2021). *International Health Regulations | IHR core capacities*. Retrieved from https://www.euro.who.int/en/health-topics/health-emergencies/international-health-regulations/capacity-building/ihr-core-capacities

Zanluca, C., De Melo, V. C. A., Mosimann, A. L. P., Dos Santos, G. I. V., dos Santos, C. N. D., & Luz, K. (2015). First report of autochthonous transmission of Zika virus in Brazil. *Memorias Do Instituto Oswaldo Cruz, 110*(4), 569–572. https://doi.org/10.1590/0074-02760150192

Zilla, C. (2020). *Corona crisis and political confrontation in Brazil: The president, the people, and democracy under pressure* (Vol. 36). Stiftung Wissenschaft Und Politik -SWP- Deutsches Institut Für Internationale Politik Und Sicherheit. https://doi.org/10.18449/2020C36

Chapter 3
Community Engagement in Disease Outbreak Preparedness and Response: Lessons from Recent Outbreaks, Key Concepts, and Quality Standards for Practice

Sharon Abramowitz and Jamie Bedson

Contents

Introduction

The critical importance of putting communities at the center of public health emergencies and disease outbreak and response has garnered increased recognition in government, development, public health, and humanitarian communities. Despite four decades of efforts to define the essential role of community engagement, it is the myriad lessons emerging from the 2014–2016 Ebola Outbreak in West Africa Ebola, followed by the Zika outbreak, Ebola outbreaks in the Democratic Republic of the Congo (DRC), and the COVID-19 pandemic, that have sharpened focus on the centrality of communities in response and preparedness in public health emergencies.

S. Abramowitz
Center for Global Health Science and Security, Georgetown University, Washington, DC, USA

J. Bedson (✉)
Jamie Bedson Consulting, Seattle, WA, USA

E. Manoncourt et al. (eds.), *Communication and Community Engagement in Disease Outbreaks*, https://doi.org/10.1007/978-3-030-92296-2_3

The chapter describes the development and content of the UNICEF's Minimum Quality Standards and Indicators for Community Engagement (hereafter, "the Minimum Standards"), including a summary of literature review, conducted by the authors, focusing on the design, practice, and measurement of community engagement. Here, we draw out the key concepts, definitions, and approaches underpinning community engagement; describe the process and outcomes of drawing on lessons from recent outbreaks; and review global practice and available evidence. We use the Minimum Standards as a framework to discuss recent Ebola and COVID-19 outbreaks and assess progress toward greater integration and application of community engagement in and for epidemics. Finally, we address priority areas to improve the quality, harmonization, accountability, and optimization of community engagement.

Critical Role of Community Engagement

Community engagement is a critical component of international development and humanitarian assistance. It has been widely studied in the context of education, public health systems, and epidemic and emergency response systems. Community engagement approaches work with communities by supporting them to take their own action to address their most pressing issues. It is characterized by its commitment to grassroots participation, protection of the most vulnerable, and empowerment of local communities, all of which are reflected in the human-rights-based approaches under which the United Nations (UN) and its partners operate (UNHCR, 2008; OCHA, 2018; Ackerman Gulaid & Kiragu, 2012; Bonelli et al., 2014).

Community engagement is critical for empowering communities, community leaders, and community organizations to play a role in improving the equity and impact of the government, development, and humanitarian initiatives that affect them. Community engagement is critical in that it aims to ensure that:

- Communities are meaningful stakeholders in two-way, transparent, and open flows of information. Preparedness and response mechanisms are in place to sustain two-way communication.
- Communities are supported to know and claim their rights. They have meaningful ownership and leadership roles in the deliberations, decision-making, design, implementation, and measurement of actions that affect them.
- Community diversity is reflected in participatory processes without discrimination, including gender, ability, age, faith, race, ability, and ethnicity.
- Community-based power inequalities are addressed, not reinforced, through community engagement actions.
- Communities have mechanisms to register concerns and provide continuous feedback on the quality, availability, accessibility, and acceptability of services. This feedback is listened to, and appropriate responses are taken.

- Programs, projects, and policies are adapted to and aligned with the needs, priorities, values, and cultures of local populations.
- Programs, projects, and policies are adapted to and aligned with the needs, priorities, and policies of national, sub-national, and local governments.
- The quality of research, evaluation, and monitoring of community engagement is tied to community structures, processes, and ownership, so that communities have influence over research documenting the issues that impact them (UNICEF, 2020).

While the centrality of community engagement is well recognized, until recently, there were no efforts to develop commonly understood international standards for designing, implementing, supporting, coordinating, integrating, resourcing, and measuring community engagement. Thus, achieving these ends, and measuring progress toward them, has been an ongoing challenge.

While there is a clear consensus that engaging with communities is critical for effective health emergency preparedness and response, there has been ambiguity about whether community engagement is a means to an end, or an end in itself. This has implications for how community engagement approaches and measurement are viewed and utilized by governments, humanitarian organizations, and within the context of preparedness and response.

The challenges associated with improving the quality, accountability, harmonization, and optimization of community engagement into public health responses can focus issues related to:

1. The methodologies and approaches utilized across contexts and how these are coordinated and integrated into responses.
2. Research and measurement of community engagement of community enragement, including understanding "what works."

Overview of the Literature

The authors conducted literature reviews of the "gray literature" (nongovernmental organization [NGO] and technical reports), peer-reviewed research, international guidance documents, and international standards and accords, with a focus on the principles underpinning community engagement, the practice of community engagement and its effectiveness, impact, research, and lessons learned. These reviews were conducted as part of two initiatives: (1) the development of the *Minimum Quality Standards and Indicators for Community Engagement* undertaken for UNICEF (JB and SA); and (2) the development of the ELRHA-supported research project "Humanizing the design of the Ebola response in DRC: anthropological research on humane designs of Ebola treatment and care to build trust for better health" conducted in North Kivu, DRC, from 2019 to 2020 under principal investigators Sung-Joon Park and Nene Morisho (SA).

Key Concepts

The history of community engagement precedes the evolution of the technical term "community engagement." Historically, some of the key conceptual principles of community engagement have been captured under the domain of participatory appraisal and participatory development.[1] As such, the basic definitional criteria for community engagement are difficult to determine. A realist review identified the following common themes that persist across multiple statements of community engagement principles: "Ensure staff provide supportive and facilitative leadership to citizens based on transparency; foster a safe and trusting environment enabling citizens to provide input; ensure citizens' early involvement; share decision-making and governance control with citizens; acknowledge and address citizens' experiences of power imbalances between citizens and professionals; invest in citizens who feel they lack the skills and confidence to engage; create quick and tangible wins; take into account both citizens' and organizations' motivations."[6]

It is challenging to develop definitions for community engagement. Subtle differences in the use of terms like community engagement, community mobilization, social mobilization, community capacity, community empowerment, participatory development are pervasive throughout the literature, but the phenomena they describe have considerable overlaps. Shared themes of participation, collective action, and capacity development recur in the community engagement literature. Community engagement and social mobilization is regularly defined as a "process" that is systematic and deliberate, with the corollary that the actions can be subjected to some standardization.

The UNICEF definition provided in the Minimum Standards highlights the fact that community engagement involves purposive localized action among multiple stakeholders in contexts that are stratified by inequalities in access, resources, and power. It is recommended for use in all contexts.

> ***Community Engagement:*** *A foundational action for working with traditional, community, civil society, government, and opinion groups and leaders; and expanding collective or group roles in addressing the issues that affect their lives. Community engagement empowers social groups and social networks, builds upon local strengths and capacities, and improves local participation, ownership, adaptation, and communication. Through community engagement principles and strategies, all stakeholders gain access to processes for assessing, analyzing, planning, leading, implementing, monitoring, and evaluating actions, programs, and policies that will promote survival, development, protection and participation* (UNICEF, 2020).

There is a notable distinction between academic definitions for community engagement and gray literature or programmatic approaches to community engagement. In

[1]These include Participatory Learning Action (PLA); rapid rural appraisal (RRA); Participatory Rural Appraisal (PRA); Participatory Research and Assessment (PRA); Participatory Action Research (PAR); Participatory Poverty Assessments (PPA), community/social mobilization, community participation, community capacity building, community empowerment, Communicating with Communities (CwC), and Community Engagement and Accountability (CEA).

academic work, the concept of community engagement requires the premise that communities retain the right of dissent, the right of local expertise, and the right to pursue alternative paths that contradict those offered by the program (Lavery et al., 2010). In technical and professional "gray literatures," including organizational procedural manuals and guidelines for practice, community engagement practice frequently disregards dissent or reframes dissent as an issue of "resistance," and focuses on achieving purposive community participation, compelled community participation using the influence of state structures or stakeholders, or "convincing" communities using a wide array of communications and marketing approaches. Techniques that align well with the gray literature on community engagement align well with instrumentalist practices of social mobilization—the mobilization of local communities toward a purposive end. It also aligns with behavior change communication, which highlights a targeted set of behaviors or practices that require modification for specific ends.

There is broad agreement in the literature about the fundamental principles underpinning community engagement. How principles translate into practice and programming, however, differs widely. The variation observed is associated with approaches used, degrees of participation, prioritized domains, and program objectives among other factors. The community engagement principles presented in this section drew upon existing international conventions, agreement, and standards, as well as NGO documents. They are also presumed to be the foundation of efforts taken toward achieving other international conventions, including the Sustainable Development Goals (SDGs) and the International Health Regulations (IHR) (UNDP, 2016; World Health Assembly, 2005).

Community Engagement Approaches

There are a range of community engagement approaches discussed in the practice literature. Most describe some step-by-step project cycle approaches, for example, the Community Action Cycle (Howard-Grabman & Snetro, 2015), that operate over a fixed term and follow the ubiquitous developmental or humanitarian project cycle. These approaches can be categorized into: (a) primary approaches—or specific and targeted approaches with the end goal of creating community engagement; and (b) instrumental or integrated approaches—use of community engagement approaches to achieve other ends (Howard-Grabman & Snetro, 2015; Mercy Corps, 2009).

Primary approaches to community engagement treat engagement and mobilization as an end, not a means to an end. Primary approaches implement community engagement programs that are specifically focused on mobilizing communities and on addressing issues identified by communities. These approaches often note that this approach has limited impact until community actions are integrated into existing structures, systems, clusters, and government policy and processes.

Instrumental approaches to community engagement use community engagement approaches and social mobilization methodologies to accomplish non-community engagement objectives (e.g., health, education, protection, or civil society outcomes) in a participatory and empowering manner (Howard-Grabman & Snetro, 2015; Mercy Corps, 2009).

The approaches adopted by different organizations reflect how community engagement integrates with the theory of change of respective institutions. Most approaches presume that community engagement occurs continuously in a reciprocating loop of information, feedback, consideration, and reorientation. The widely known "P Process" (Health Communications Capacity Collaborative, 2013) is best known for this kind of reciprocating feedback loop and is credited as a planned process that can be highly participatory. Community engagement processes can be systematic while also being highly participatory, flexible, adaptable, and responsive to the voices of community actors. Whether community engagement is "primary" or "instrumental," there is a pervasive lack of clarity about how to manage community engagement in coordination, and how to manage community engagement in decommissioning or handover processes when programs end. Coordination and handover are frequent blind spots in guidelines promoting long-term, "sustainable," community engagement.

Minimum Quality Standards and Indicators for Community Engagement: An Overview

In an attempt to address the gap between theory and practice in community engagement approaches and reach a foundational consensus for advancing both programming and research, an 18-month international consultation process was undertaken by UNICEF to reflect: (a) the need for developing minimum standards, including a shared language and understanding of the role of all stakeholders and how community engagement should be measured, and (b) build in the flexibility for those standards to be adapted and localized as needed.

The Minimum Standards that emerged from this process are organized into four sections and cover core standards, implementation, coordination and integration, and resource mobilization. Table 3.1 provides a summary of the Inter-Agency Minimum Quality Standards and Indicators for Community Engagement:

The rationale for the structure of the standards is to emphasize the need for a holistic understanding of the minimum requirement for community engagement activities across a series of area and to emphasize the need for it to be integrated across the humanitarian and health emergency structures.

- **Part A: Core Community Engagement Standards.** These describe the fundamental standards that should guide community engagement practice. They should be mainstreamed across all aspects of practice. They are cross-cutting and should be applied to all aspects of standards included in Parts B, C, and D.
- **Part B: Standards Supporting Implementation.** These standards are aligned to elements of the project cycle. They define the scope of practice for engaging communities. They explicitly target informed design, planning and preparation, management of activities, and monitoring and evaluation.

Table 3.1 Summary of minimum standards for community engagement

Part A: Core Community Engagement Standards	Part B: Standards Supporting Implementation
1. Participation 2. Empowerment and ownership 3. Inclusion 4. Two-way communication 5. Adaptability and localization 6. Building on local capacity	7. Informed design 8. Planning and preparation 9. Managing activities 10. Monitoring, evaluation, and learning
	Part C: Standards Supporting Coordination and Integration 11. Government leadership 12. Partner coordination 13. Integration
	Part D: Standards Supporting Resource Mobilization 14. Human resources and organizational structures 15. Data management 16. Resource mobilization and budgeting

Source: United Nations Children's Fund (UNICEF) (2020)

- **Part C: Standards Supporting Coordination and Integration.** These standards focus on supporting collective, harmonized, and mutually supportive community engagement practice at national and local levels. Coordination addresses how partners coordinate their activities with other partners, government, response clusters/pillars, and communities. It supports policy and strategy alignment and common protocols and resolves geographic and functional duplication. Integration involves the inclusion of community engagement in all aspects of development programming, governance, and humanitarian response structures, systems, policies, and plans. Governments have a primary role in leading the coordination and integration of community engagement in "peacetime" and emergency contexts.
- **Part D: Standards Supporting Resource Mobilization.** Standards supporting resource mobilization focus on key management and administrative considerations that determine quality community engagement. The resourcing of community engagement is human capital intensive and can require complex operational imperatives that involve significant budgetary consideration, like human resources, training, significant time investments, logistics, and safety and security protocols.

Progress and Challenges: Recent Outbreaks Through the Lens of the Minimum Standards

The Minimum Standards provide a framework of analysis for reviewing community engagement practice in recent health emergencies. In this section, we discuss the Ebola responses in West Africa and the DRC and consider the emerging issues related to the COVID-19 outbreak using the Minimum Standards structure (Table 3.1) as an analytical lens. We describe the requirements for specific standards, report identified gaps in practice, give examples of success, and detail recommendations and lessons for future (and ongoing) responses.

Participation

Participation in nearly all aspects of Ebola, from case identification to quarantine to the management of the bodies of the dead (Shultz et al., 2016; Nielsen et al., 2015; Nau, 2014; Richards & Fairhead, 2014; Saez & Borchert, 2014; Moran, 2017; Johnson et al., 2015; Lipton, 2014), is an essential aspect of ensuring community involvement with Ebola response activities and has been robustly documented (O'Sullivan et al., 2018). Research on "social learning" during the Liberia Ebola outbreak found that Monrovia communities were able to rapidly uptake behavior change messages, try them out, and retain those that were feasible while discarding those that were plainly not feasible, even while holding views that are commonly characterized as "rumours and misinformation" (Abramowitz et al., 2018). Detailed guidance documents and training materials on participation have been developed for field-based humanitarian actors (Groupe URD, 2009).

Empowerment and Local Ownership

Community leadership and ownership in all aspects of localized healthcare, including a One Health approach, is recognized as a fundamental norm for health systems strengthening in sub-Saharan African countries (Dickmann et al., 2018). Empowerment and local ownership are central to the successful implementation of community engagement. However, extensive anthropological documentation from the Ebola outbreaks in Sierra Leone and DRC demonstrates that there is a clear distinction between local leadership and local acceptability. Local leaders, like paramount chiefs and traditional healers, had the opportunity to manipulate and divert response resources (Le Marcis et al., 2019) forcibly coerce individuals to engage in socially and culturally unacceptable practices (Parker et al., 2019), and leverage community engagement leadership roles for alternate political agendas (Wilkinson et al., 2017). Without local buy-in or acceptance of leadership mandates, community members diverted sick family members to areas where they could provide direct care, and bury their deceased family members and friends in locations where they could be mourned (Richards, 2016; Richards et al., 2015a, b).

Inclusion

Community engagement can and should provide a mechanism for vulnerable individuals, minority groups, survivors, women, children, adolescents, and young adults (Frazer, 2019), and individuals with disabilities to access full participation in Ebola activities. Attention must be placed to ethnic, class, education, gender, and language differences among populations impacted or at risk of Ebola, as well as differences between community engagement workers and local populations (Alcayna-Stevens, 2018). This can be particularly challenging in the context of Ebola outbreaks, when engagement and empowerment with local leaders can come at the expense of the engagement and empowerment of marginalized populations. Substantial research has been dedicated to analyzing the experiences of Ebola survivors, stigmatization, and leadership and participation in Ebola response after surviving the disease (Schwerdtle et al., 2017).

Through community engagement strategies, diverse modalities of communication can reach individuals with different levels of access to information, and different levels of proximate risk. For example, one study found that women were more likely to access information about Ebola through household-based sensitization activities and familial and social networks, while men had more access to information through radio and cell phones (Kangbai, 2016). Other studies found that men and women had different (even if numerically equivalent) pathways to exposure based on their social roles, with women providing primary caregiving to individuals in the household, and men providing care and transportation in the community (Abramowitz et al., 2015; Nkangu et al., 2017). A deeper dive on gender is warranted (see also Oxfam's report (Carter et al., 2017)), but it is important to note that the qualitative data on gender from the North Kivu epidemic vastly exceeds the quality of data collected during the West Africa Ebola epidemic.

Two-Way Communication

Risk communications have historically been privileged by the World Health Organization as the dominant modality for reaching populations during epidemic outbreaks. Risk communications—with an emphasis on mass media, uniform, and sanctioned government and response messaging, and the public distribution of information materials—have historically prioritized "one-way" communications infrastructures that push information out from a technical leadership core.

This bias toward mass communications persisted into the West Africa Ebola outbreak (Storey et al., 2017), delaying robust investment in a two-way communications infrastructure based on community engagement with widely documented disastrous results (Wilkinson et al., 2017; Chandler et al., 2015; McGovern, 2014). These included the inappropriate stigmatization of bushmeat, massive, and media-based fear-mongering that inhibited participation in response activities and utilization of response services like Ebola treatment units (ETUs) and militarized national and international responses using security forces from developed countries (UK and US) which further terrified local populations and lead to the concealment of cases, resistance, and non-response to intervention mechanisms (Hoffman, 2016; Heymann, 2017). Messages distributed through one-way communication systems also seem to have been incapable of addressing core challenges around mistrust and misinformation.

Adaptability and Localization

There are many kinds of communities, each with their own histories and their own socio-cultural, political, migration, economic, structural, and geographical characteristics. The range of communities, and the immense social flux that characterizes them, makes communities uniquely significant potential frontline responders to epidemics. Building local community engagement infrastructure, however, is notoriously difficult due to problems with scaling uniform models into diverse settings. Local adaptations are needed when community engagement approaches are scaled to new regions, contexts, and sectors (Ottolenghi et al., 2018; Tedrow et al., 2012).

Typically, however, adaptability and localization have been treated as an afterthought in the community engagement technical literature. Guidelines are offered on best practices, ethics, and procedures, with a caveat at the beginning or the end of a technical guidance indicating that community engagement should be localized and adapted to local populations. The meta-analyses and literature reviews above all consistently demonstrate that localization and adaptation are required for successful community engagement; they also note that because localization and adaptation occur, comparability between sites is very difficult to achieve, and successful programs are enormously difficult to replicate and measure.

It seems, therefore, that the practice of adaptability and localization itself is a part of the core suite of community engagement interventions that must occur. By taking the time to understand, analyze, and communicate with local communities sufficiently deeply that meaningful adaptability and localization occur, community-level workers do critical political and discursive work that enables subsequent uptake in Ebola prevention and response practices, and identify local networks and capacities to build into a localized prevention and response architecture.

Building on Local Capacity

Extensive research has demonstrated that communities have impressive indigenous protocols, practices, languages, and procedures for addressing disease outbreak. Frederic Le Marcis has called indigenous responses to epidemic outbreaks "social immunization" (Le Marcis, 2016) and is currently conducting extensive research on local languages and practices that preexisted Ebola that were used to respond to Ebola outbreaks in Guinea's Forestiére communities. Research in Uganda, DRC (Hewlett & Hewlett, 2007), and Sierra Leone (Richards, 2016) has shown that communities have developed approaches for restricting mobility to prevent disease spread, isolation and quarantine, positioning disease survivors as caretakers, abstention from sexual relations, managing burials, and caregiving practices for the sick that are grounded in local languages, religions, cultural practices, norms, and values.

Community engagement, at its best, engages widely trusted interlocutors to help institutions tap into these localized networks and capacities, and leverage them for prevention, infection prevention and control (IPC), treatment, and safe and dignified burials. More typically, however, community engagement and social mobilization are tied to the adoption of novel or unique capacities for incident reporting, contact tracing, or case identification, for example, use of the 117 phone line and community event-based surveillance (CEBS) systems in Sierra Leone (Alpren et al., 2017; Larsen et al., 2017). Local capacity requires the mobilization of latent social structures, systems, and resources for community engagement purposes to prevent and respond to disease outbreaks. Qualitative research and community engagement data collection found that in partnership with community engagement, the imposition of by-laws by Sierra Leone's paramount chiefs, limitations on mobility through the use of voluntary roadblocks, and close proximate access to high quality care were effective in limiting transmission (Gray et al., 2018).

Building on local capacity means recognizing and leveraging the fact that traditional healers (Manguvo & Mafuvadze, 2015), midwives (Schwartz et al., 2019), pharmacists (Wilkinson et al., 2014), and burial experts (Moran, 2017) continue to provide care for the sick and the dying using the best information available to them at the time. Incidents of these persons as having expand the epidemic through massive local transmission events have been circulated widely (McNeil, 2014), but the implications of the widespread nature of these practices have not been translated into the model for community engagement that is currently conceptualized in Ebola response as focused on "risk communications." Building on local capacity will require improving the capacity of community engagement workers to identify and engage with the sociocultural, health, and physical ecologies of local communities, so that Ebola responses are grounded in core local strengths and capacities. In Ebola outbreaks, building on local capacity also means recognizing that Ebola survivors are more than passive victims. It is vital to mobilize survivor groups for community engagement, social mobilization, and other response activities (Lee-Kwan et al., 2014).

Implementation

If the Core Community Engagement Standards set forth the "why" of community engagement, Implementation details the "who, what, where, and when." However, the literature on implementation is plagued by fundamental disagreements in each of these areas.

- For "Who?": Are implementors the persons responsible for grassroots interventions? Program supervisors? Program designers? Community leaders? Community members? Donors? State Actors? Or some networked aggregation of all these stakeholders?
- For "What?": Is community engagement Implementation a set of principles, practices, or programs? Is it tools, techniques, methods, or relationships? Is it associated with processes or outcomes?
- For "Where": Is community engagement's site the geographic locus of the problem (e.g., an area affected by a spreading disease)? Is it the social network impacted by the intervention? Is it the local physical space in which community engagement occurs? Is it the intended geopolitical region predicted to be impacted by community engagement practices?
- For "When": Is community engagement a teleological process that moves community actors from "unlearned" to "learned?" Is it a program cycle that begins with conceptualization, funding, and planning; reaches its fulcrum in "implementation," and is then monitored and evaluated to deduce lessons learned? Or is community engagement's timeline tied to longer term trajectories for development and governance systems?

None of these questions have easy answers and vary widely by context, condition, and intent. In recent years, countries affected by Ebola have mobilized community engagement through "who's". These are typically international donors and program managers who work through local networks of employees and volunteers to "sensitize" local populations to Ebola-related concerns. The "what" has typically included the transfer of information regarding the Ebola virus disease, the international response, clinical trials, emergency response mechanisms like hotline numbers, and information about services, healing, and triage. In some contexts, like Sierra Leone in 2014–2015, the "what" has also included the development of a community plans to "triggers" localized response measures to protect the community from Ebola, and expedite response if disease is detected. The "where" has included villages, towns, and cities affected by Ebola cases, and neighboring regions (including cross-border areas) that were identified as being at high risk; and needed to take preventive measures. Community engagement has tended to be highly localized, and coordination, when it occurs, has occurred at the sub-national level.

Of all these, the "when" has been most problematic. Community engagement during an Ebola response has frequently been tied to post-outbreak timeframes; when the emergence of widespread fear,[43] sufficient to impact other operational responses, and manifestations of "community resistance" create difficulties for the mobilization of other response priorities. There are other ways to frame the "when" in community engagement implementation. Ideally, community engagement should be always mainstreamed into national, sub-national, and local public sector capacities for the surveillance of and response to critical events, and to the execution of routine community mobilization activities. These capacities can be embedded into national health and educational systems. For zoonotic diseases like Ebola, however, community engagement capacities should be embedded into One Health-guided systems that take an ecological approach to human and animal interaction and can rapidly identify and respond to the human and animal dimensions of Ebola transmission, as close to the site of zoonotic "leaps" from human to animal as possible (Quammen, 2014).

Informed Design

Informed design involves pre-research—particularly qualitative and anthropological research—on the conditions that will impact community engagement. In contexts affected by Ebola, this means that designers of community engagement initiatives need to have a comprehensive understanding of the local social, economic, political, health, and governance contexts. A realistic understanding of institutional and community capacity for implementation is also crucial. In the context of Ebola outbreaks in Sub-Saharan Africa, for example, it is essential that community engagement programs take into account local attitudes toward governance, security, surveillance, and public health interventions (Hofman & Au, 2017; Heymann et al., 2015). It requires that people take all necessary steps to understand local cosmologies and explanatory models for disease origins, disease transmission, disease treatment, and public health containment, including how local populations understand the spiritual and political implications of the disease and its impact on caregivers, survivors, and family members of infected persons (Hewlett & Hewlett, 2007; Hewlett & Amola, 2003; Hewlett et al., 2005). Frequently, as Barry Hewlett found in Uganda and Frederic Le Marcis found in Guinea, traditional knowledge includes essential and accurate linguistic, medical, and public health knowledges that are effective at characterizing Ebola disease in a way that allows the communities to contain or stop the spread of the virus (Quammen, 2014).

Planning and Preparation

The practitioner literature nearly always stipulates that meaningful qualitative research[60] and localized community participation are necessary for community engagement planning and preparation (UNHCR, 2008). Planning and preparation, at a minimum, involves establishing contact, identifying stakeholders from a wide range of social, cultural, political, and economic locations, conducting an initial in-person assessment (which involves introducing oneself and creating a space for exchange), analyzing the context using a holistic approach, and analyzing and discussing needs and demands with local populations. Médecins Sans Frontières' (MSF) Vienna Evaluation Unit developed detailed guidance for understanding communities, negotiating community entry, and using medical anthropological approaches in initial engagement with local communities (Medécins Sans Frontièrs, 2013). Importantly, MSF's work also aligns qualitative methodologies with the program cycle that is often deployed in health emergency response: assessment, establishing contact with the community, participatory project design, implementing the project, monitoring and evaluation, and exit strategy (ibid, 2013).

Building upon these activities, best practices call for the development of a partnership agreement with the local communities, and laying the groundwork for participatory project design, implementation, and evaluation.

Managing Activities

Managing activities involves the execution of the activities determined during planning and preparation phases. It also involves the identification and mobilization of human, material, and service resources, sustaining active two-way communication pathways, and continuous monitoring to assess activity suitability, progress, and planning appropriateness (and make changes when needed).

Community engagement is routinely called upon to execute tasks of social mobilization like door-to-door household visits, community meetings, surveys, and task-related projects. People who do community engagement, however, are often called upon to do more than just the work of community engagement. Through the work of community engagement, they are involved in tasks directly associated with surveillance, contact tracing, trainings, provision of care in clinical and non-clinical contexts, supporting quarantine, case identification, and coordination and negotiation with local leaders. At the level of program design, community involvement in the development of community action plans was a fundamental feature of Social Mobilization Action Consortium's (SMAC) (Bedson et al., 2020) activities in Sierra Leone; but it was less pronounced in Liberia's and Guinea's experiences, where community engagement was based on a social mobilization model that implicated a grassroots approach to mass communication, rather than deliberative process.

Sustaining a dialogue between external community engagement actors, local community engagement actors, and communities is essential for success. Sustaining dialogue, however, is more often an ideal than a reality in many community engagement approaches, due to under-investment in community engagement systems capacities. It also invites the opportunity for interactions that community engagement leaders may find uncomfortable, including questioning, reluctance, resistance, and refusal.

Monitoring, Evaluation, and Learning

Community engagement can and has been measured, at-scale, in the context of health emergencies. Mass interventions during the recent West African Ebola and Zika outbreaks have collected both process and behavioral intentions data and demonstrated the "possible" for future responses. Key to data collection within the context of these interventions is in ensuring that the collection of data was fully integrated into interventions and that tools for collection and analysis were placed in the hands of mobilizers and communities.

Community engagement is deeply connected to participatory approaches to monitoring, evaluation, and learning in Ebola outbreaks and beyond (Munodawafa et al., 2018). Fundamentally, monitoring and evaluation involve the movement of information; and that is based on the core implementation of community engagement practices, systems, and capabilities. Some would go so far as to say that building a participatory monitoring and evaluation system is a constitutive part of community engagement, while others would question the necessity of these measures in the context of public health and humanitarian emergencies.

There is insufficient evidence to determine whether any particular practice, model, or approach is more effective than others (O'Mara-Eves et al., 2015; Popay et al., 2007), but wide and unexplained variation in was reported in some studies (Azad et al., 2010; Tripathy et al., 2010). There is no "one-size-fits-all" approach for any particular model of community engagement (McCoy et al., 2012; Victora & Barros, 2013).

The evidence base quantifying the impacts of community engagement within the context of health emergencies is slight, making it difficult for policy makers, funding agencies and humanitarian actors to determine how to allocate resources and integrate community engagement interventions into response operations. This being the case, there is a broader—though not comprehensive—evidence base on the development sector from which lessons can and should be drawn to inform future responses. Participants agreed that having more rigorous evidence on community engagement interventions will contribute to improving practice and resource allocation across the sector.

There is great scope for the social science and epidemiology/modeling communities to intensify collaboration Abramowitz et al. (2017). Mathematical modeling experts noted that the assumptions about human behavior made in mathematical disease models typically do not draw on the deep knowledge about people and cultures that exists within the social sciences. Social science practitioners noted that more modeling of social data may offer considerable opportunity to test hypotheses and better analyze existing data. Work is needed to reach common ground and improve methodological approaches amongst epidemiological modelers, social scientists and RCCE practitioners (Bedson et al., 2021).

Modeling of social interventions in an epidemic is limited by a lack of reliable, at-scale field data collection on social and behavioral indicators, along with indicators that measure the process of community engagement. The need for homogeneous guidelines and standardized indicators and approaches for data collection is needed to enable modeling and measurement across contexts. Such guidelines could include how to establish a social behavior baseline, including geospatial factors of transmission, in addition to setting requirements for establishing a stable record of data sets and how they were collected. Implementing agencies, including governments and NGO practitioners, often have deep knowledge and collect substantial amounts of data on local community responses. However, due to a lack of capacity, time, funding, or mandate for undertaking further research and analysis, this data may remain on a shelf without being analyzed or published. Better linkages between practitioners and academics, and between qualitative and quantitative research communities, can help to bring this data to light for further analysis and publication.

There is a significant evidence gap related to the relative efficacy of financing community engagement as compared to other interventions.

Coordination and Integration

The West Africa Ebola response was characterized by a deep reluctance to organize the massive and systematic community engagement response needed to slow down or end the epidemic (Laverack & Manoncourt, 2016). According to one article written by principals involved with the response, this epidemic was the first time that UNICEF Communications for Development (C4D) was asked to lead an independent response pillar (cluster) that focused on social mobilization and community engagement (Gillespie et al., 2016). These actors found that they were able to distill seven key lessons from the experience:

1. Strategy and decentralization (including adequate funding, supplies for decentralized tasks) were necessary for successful community engagement.
2. Coordination of community engagement, including the development of standard operating procedures (SOPs), was necessary to ensure timely and relevant community engagement interventions.
3. Entering and engaging communities required trust. Close associations with entities like community care centers, schools, and survivor groups had trust-building impacts for the entirety of the response.
4. Messaging needed to be continually adjusted to respond to changing levels of knowledge exposure among the general population, and new requirements for information.
5. Broad partnerships with multiple actors were essential, including with religious leaders and local journalists and media.
6. Management and capacity building (training and supervision) was necessary to ensure quality community engagement.
7. The Ebola epidemic presented an opportunity to innovate in data collection, research, and measurement of community engagement[72] (ibid, 2016).

During the COVID-19 outbreak, this need for greater coordination has resulted in the establishment of the Risk Communication and Community Engagement Collective Service, a partnership between UNICEF, WHO, and International Federation of Red Cross and Red Crescent Societies (IFRC). Efforts such as this reflect a view of community enragement as an approach that requires not only shared standards and measurement but also ongoing and iterative use of shared data, efforts to address systemic barriers to community engagement coordination and integration, and a shared purpose between organizations that are often working in parallel (or at its worst competing) within the humanitarian space.

Government Leadership

In West Africa, government leadership in community engagement coordination varied widely in each of the three most affected countries (Hansch et al., 2018). In Liberia, community engagement and social mobilization were prioritized at the peak of the outbreak, and was closely integrated into the incident management system (IMS) structure that was directly (and strongly) led by the Liberian government (Nyenswah, 2017). After the epidemic peaked, community engagement was integrated into the "ring approach." This was a rapid response mechanism that surged all pillar capacities within communities during reported outbreaks simultaneously, and with great intensity (Nyenswah et al., 2015, 2016; Kateh et al., 2015; Lindblade et al., 2015). In Sierra Leone, community engagement was largely implemented by a coalition of organizations called the Social Mobilization Action Committee (SMAC) (Pedi et al., 2017; Bedson et al., 2020; SMAC, 2014), which worked under the National Ebola Response Centre (NERC) and the District Ebola Response Centres (DERCs) in a "hybrid model" with the government to direct community engagement activities in more than 10,000 communities. In Guinea, community engagement coordination was introduced very late, and in an ad hoc fashion, through independent organizations responding to the epidemic, but centralized coordination was weak and government involvement was highly politicized.

Nyenswah, one of the key leaders of the Liberia response, highlighted the following government leadership requirements for a successful response:

- There is no substitute for strong political leadership.
- To lead effectively, there must be a strong supporting cast.
- Governments must take ownership of the response.
- Systems and structures must be put into place early by the government.
- Relationships with international partners must be managed well.
- Leadership comes from within, but opportunities to lead come from outside.
- Mistakes will be made, and it is important to learn from them (Nyenswah, 2017).

Several memoirs have demonstrated that the lack of government leadership is widely perceived as having created chaotic and ineffective response environments in both Guinea and Sierra Leone (Walsh & Johnson, 2018). In Guinea, community engagement leaders conducted research and identified that there was a learning curve for governments and response actors. Early on, they note that "communities were initially subjected to coercive methods of prevention and control of Ebola and were stigmatized. This context subsequently led to two forms of resistance from communities in relation to the actors of prevention: passive and active resistance." This unfavorable approach was ultimately abandoned in favor of an active (but decentralized) community engagement and community involvement approach that contributed to the end of the epidemic (Mamadou Mbaye et al., 2017).

There is a contradictory interpretation of the role of governments in Ebola-related community engagement, which views community engagement through the lens of neoliberal reforms, postcolonial inequality, and government distrust (Benton & Dionne, 2015). In this view, social mobilization and community engagement are mobilized to function as a kind of "alt-state" that solely exists to address the problem of Ebola. As a dozen contributors make clear in their contributions to Ibrahim Abdallah and Ismail Rashid's book *Understanding West Africa's Ebola Epidemic: Towards a Political Economy*, massive social mobilization is required to respond to Ebola when government systems are structured to be weak and ineffective; or where governments are widely mistrusted, struggle with corruption and abuse, and fail to encourage and sustain widespread political engagement (Abdullah & Rashid, 2017). Here, community engagement is represented as the antithesis of failed governance. It can be interpreted as the grassroots construction of ad hoc "governance" through the rapid rollout of information through latent social networks. Or alternately, community engagement and social mobilization fulfill a self-fulfilling prophecy of "failed statehood" by functioning as a last line of defense when weak states prove ineffective at fulfilling core functions. At the same time, community engagement fulfills a built-in design flaw in poor and marginalized countries that requires that governments function ineffectively, and always require external assistance, but especially during times of crisis.

Following the West Africa Ebola outbreak, there has been an explosion of calls to mainstream communities into health systems strengthening (HSS); this requires the national governmental prioritization of community engagement capacities for planning and priority-setting; program implementation; monitoring, evaluation, and quality improvement; and advocacy (Sacks et al., 2017). Communities create an "enabling" environment and play an "enabling role" in this construction (ibid, 2017). There is a growing sense that community engagement is the missing leg in global public health. Preparedness for epidemics—a key feature of HSS approaches—requires investments in durable community-based infrastructure that can be rapidly mobilized and scaled at the time of outbreaks (Tambo et al., 2017; Heymann et al., 2015). West Africa's experience shows that while partner commitments to long-term investments are extended during epidemics; follow through is compromised by significant global political, financial, and structural factors (Ravi et al., 2019).

National governments must lead in epidemic coordination; they are indispensable actors (Piot et al., 2019). Only national governments can ensure long-term commitments to laboratory capacity, community engagement capacity, surveillance systems, and quality clinical care. Each of these commitments have direct implications for the integration of community engagement in EVD response capacity. Anthropologists have repeatedly noted that the centralization of response authority in governments that may have a history of violence and abuse toward local populations is ineffective and alienates local communities (Enria et al., 2016). This is fully accurate, and governments must lead from a place of core commitment to human rights.

Partner Coordination

Under WHO epidemic response leadership, community engagement, and partner coordination has been a weakness in the mobilization of Ebola response activities (Frieden, 2018). We learned from the UN Mission for Ebola Emergency Response (UNMEER) experience that partner coordination, when convened at too high a level, for too short a period of time, with insufficient buy-in from stakeholders can divert attention and resources and undermine national authority in the response. Community engagement is a clear area in which these gaps are evident, particularly in the North Kivu response. However, the establishment of the Risk Communication and Community Engagement Collective Service points to a potentially new era of coordination between key international actors. The sharing and joint consolidation of data and subsequent planning is much needed at all levels of response - community, national, regional and international.

Integration

Community engagement continues to be treated as a capacity that is quite apart from core response capacities like case identification and contact tracing, despite significant evidence suggesting that community engagement is a core part of both case identification and contact tracing in "real world" situations (Abramowitz et al., 2015, 2016; Bedson et al., 2020). Individuals who are "doing" community engagement are also doing contact tracing, social mobilization, case identification, IPC training, and many other tasks in local communities (Miller et al., 2018), but they are not recognized as playing these multiple overlapping roles by response actors. Research on how contact tracing and case identification works at the local level, how community-level workers are integrated into those processes, and to what extent novel data collection tools are convenient and effective are in their infancy (Larsen et al., 2017). Further work is needed to systematize the integration community engagement into case identification and contact tracing capabilities (Houlihan et al., 2017), but when this was practiced in Liberia, successful results were observed (Sepers et al., 2019).

Additionally, community engagement capacity needs to be integrated into humanitarian response mechanisms in order to ensure that the rapid deployment of community engagement systems is not delayed by failures to take into account local security contexts (Mobula et al., 2018). As noted by key social scientist observers, this creates sometimes untenable dialectical pressures between risk and proximity, distance and contact that creates unbearable burdens for responders and community members alike (Enria, 2019). This is the needle that must be threaded with care, patience, and continual effort. Historically, public health risk communications had no tradition of working in partnership with humanitarian response capabilities; this was recognized as a priority for change in post-Ebola reflection pieces from West Africa. However, long delays in the mobilization of community engagement capacities due to local security concerns, and failures to activate international humanitarian security capabilities to facilitate community engagement, directly lead to the systematic delays and under-development of community engagement capabilities in North Kivu.

Resource Mobilization

Community engagement—as an action—has not been sufficient in Ebola response contexts. A full complement of supporting capabilities is required to ensure that community engagement has the "staff, stuff, and systems" needed to ensure effective integration. Efforts were made to document community engagement systems during the West Africa Ebola epidemic in the hopes that these would be scaled across epidemic preparedness and response efforts in the long-term. While promising, continued resourcing and prioritization is needed for COVID-19 and other future disease response.

Human Resources and Organizational Structures

Community engagement needs to be recognized as a specific skill set that requires training, support, supervision, and compensation. While in a surge environment, individuals can be trained rapidly to participate or lead short-term community engagement activities, effectiveness is substantially supported by the presence of standard operating procedures, institutional structures, and dedicated capacities. In Sierra Leone, the SMAC coalition used the Water, Sanitation, and Hygiene (WASH) template for community-lead total sanitation (CLTS) to design Community-led Ebola Action (CLEA) (SMAC, 2014) methodology and contribute to the development nationwide community engagement SOPs (Pedi et al., 2017). Minimum standards, national and international guidelines, and Terms of Reference (TORs) should all be pre-positioned for rapid deployment. Given the widespread acceptance of CLTS in the WASH community, WASH actors working in Ebola environments are frequently early adopters and supporters for community engagement.

By prioritizing an emphasis on human resources, this review forces the question: Is community engagement supportive of other core functions like surveillance, case identification, infection, prevention and control (IPC), care delivery, and contact tracing? Or is it physically embedded in the same persons as the individuals who are responsible in formal and informal roles for the management of all those tasks? Community engagement is a form of skilled labor. Current systems for Ebola response recognize neither the labor nor the laborer in configurations of response.

The repeated building and dismantling of extensively developed community engagement systems in the healthcare sector, just for the purpose of addressing a single disease, does a disservice to the communities who require long-term community engagement infrastructure. It is also arguably a waste of human resources, in that it trains and supports skilled workers and then abandons them without career paths; tells skilled workers that they should switch from funded to voluntary labor; and redirects motivated organizers with active social and political capital from health activities back to the private sector for livelihoods and income generation (Abramowitz et al., 2016). More than once, pay differentials have impacted the ability of healthcare workers to be able to participate in Ebola response activities with a sense that they are being treated fairly and honestly (McMahon et al., 2007).

Data Management

As indicated earlier, there is a lack of quality quantitative, qualitative, and mixed-methods empirical data to inform conclusions about the effectiveness of community engagement in international development and global health research (Popay et al., 2007; Tindana et al., 2007; Wallerstein & Duran, 2010; Marston et al., 2013; Bedson et al., 2021; Milton et al., 2012). Too often, in Ebola contexts, data collected from Knowledge, Attitudes, and Practice (KAP) surveys have substituted for a meaningful quantitative and qualitative understanding of community engagement needs, dynamics, practices, and impacts. It is not unreasonable to expect that KAP data can provide some insight into baseline mass communications messages, operational priorities, and allocation of resources, but it is often insufficient for addressing the complexity of community engagement informational and sociocultural contextual demands. But routinely, the implementation of community engagement measures is delayed due to donor and government anticipation of the results of KAP studies; leading to excessive and unnecessary delays in baseline health promotion that is urgently needed to advance prevention.

Community engagement is also increasingly being used as a mechanism for primary data capture for a range of public health research activities, but it continues to be under-invested in as a site for data collection, which limits its capacity to carry out this scope of work properly and with fidelity.

The lack of data on community engagement has been a continual bane to efforts to scale the domain for epidemic response. New research forthcoming from the Sierra Leone epidemic is demonstrating how collecting community engagement data at scale can lead to the identification of fundamental dynamics driving epidemic spread and containment (Bedson et al., 2020).

Resource Mobilization and Budgeting

Funds and budgets must be established for the rapid mobilization of community engagement capacities in future epidemics. The West Africa Ebola outbreak clearly demonstrated that community engagement systems create core capacity for long-term public health campaigns (e.g., the Global Health Security Agenda (Armstrong-Mensah & Ndiaye, 2018), universal health coverage (Odugleh-Kolev & Parrish-Sprowl, 2018), disease eradication campaigns (Baltzell et al., 2019), vaccination campaigns (Bedford et al., 2017), non-Ebola outbreak response (Nagbe et al., 2019), and clinical trials (Callis et al., 2018)), but in order to do so, they must be sustained and supported.

Moving Forward: The Standards in Practice and into the Future

The centrality of community engagement, risk communication, and other community-centered approaches is increasingly prominent with global guidance and strategy for development, health emergencies, and other humanitarian response. Whether within the SDGs setting targets for global progress, the Sphere Standards guiding humanitarian action, the Grand Bargain commitments guiding donor and aid provision, the Sendai Framework for Disaster Risk Reduction 2015–2030, placing community perspectives, action, and capacities at the center of preparedness, response and recovery is a prominent theme.

However, the COVID-19 pandemic has demonstrated that there remains significant way to go in developing the systems, strategy, budgets, and coordination required for large-scale and holistic community engagement. This is reflected in examples such as the limited number of countries that established community engagement plans for COVID-19 (Gilmore et al., 2020).

Turning the rhetoric of global guidance into action and impact with greater consistency and on a larger scale will require the continued development of tools and approaches that can align and integrate community engagement within broader response mechanisms. While a focus on key principles such as participation and inclusion are essential, these key principles will only be achieved within continued progress on standardizing measurably successful approaches, coordination at global, regional, and national level, integration of community engagement perspectives and approaches across all biomedical pillars and resources—financial, human, and technical—to achieve these goals. Mechanisms for multidisciplinary evaluation of community engagement approaches will also be essential.

As the Minimum Standards make clear, the context of any humanitarian action will ultimately guide how community engagement approaches are designed, implemented, and evaluated. While the argument of there being no "one-size-fits-all" has been employed to argue against efforts to standardize community engagement, this argument does not pass muster when held against loud and continued international calls for strong, more accountable, and more measurable community engagement. Just as biomedical approaches to diagnostics, case management, vaccine delivery is contextual depending on the disease at hand and context within which disease is being transmitted, they are equally subject to fundamental medical and technical necessities that need to be adapted. The same must be applied to community engagement. As such, the Minimum Quality Standards and Indicators for Community Engagement are not intended as a prescription intended for universal application. However, they offer a framework for, among other things: development of risk communication and community engagement (RCCE) strategy (e.g., the COVID-19 Global RCCE Strategy (WHO, 2020)), program design and implementation, holistic evaluation across a range of metrics, a checklist for donors and funders seeking to invest in community engagement activities, and a tool for identifying key skills areas in human resource management.

The Role of Key Stakeholders

Progress in taking the essential steps necessary in taking community engagement forward will be dependent on all humanitarian preparedness and response actors: (a) recognizing that community engagement is fundamental to all aspects of a health emergency from the very beginning; (b) speaking the same language and sharing a frame of reference for what approaches and measures and being utilized across institutions and in any given context; (c) understanding their role and comparative advantage in supporting an enabling environment for community engagement. This includes the utilization of internationally agreed standards across key health emergencies actors.

- *Governments:* The primary goal is to create a sustainable, durable public engagement structure that can serve as a platform for community dialogues, triggering community action, and facilitating community participation and two-way communications. On a country-by-country basis, the standards and indicators should be used to identify legislation, policies, and procedures that intersect with core aspects of community engagement implementation (e.g., risk communication, public engagement, national and local surveys, and censuses). Governments should be supported to working to change policy to support the engagement of local communities through the development of a sustainable community engagement architecture. This requires the delegation of consultation to local governments and local groups.
- *Multilateral organizations:* Community engagement is strongly associated with all aspects of effective healthcare access and delivery in emergency and development contexts. Strengthening health systems requires the institutionalization of a robust community engagement policy infrastructure, programming, human resources, and programming resource mobilization. Multilateral institutions play a lead role in establishing policy, setting standards for development and humanitarian practice, support to and coordination of governments, the private and non-governmental organization, advocacy for development and humanitarian response and directing funding to partners. As such, they are essential partners in setting international community engagement norms. Community engagement

coordination mechanisms and approaches are central to epidemic preparedness and response, and humanitarian emergencies. Increasingly, global climate change preparedness efforts are aligning, with these approaches by recognizing the importance of community resilience and local systems strengthening as a leading-edge priority for climate change resilience strategies.

- *NGOs:* Nongovernmental organizations that implement community engagement programming are key leaders for establishing norms and practices for community engagement. Implementing agencies are accountable to the communities and governments they serve. However, NGOs have their own mandates, missions, methodologies, and objectives for working with communities in development and emergency response programming. These need to be highly adaptive, context specific, and are subject to considerable resource constraints. The capacity of busy and low-resourced organizations in adapting, adopting, and implementing novel international standards should be recognized and incorporated into all efforts to establish community engagement norms. As such, it is essential that adequate resources, tools, and support be provided to enable implementing partners to utilize the standards.
- *Funding agencies:* Funding and donor agencies will play a leading role in ensuring the dissemination and adoption of the Minimum Standards. There has been robust support among partners in the consultation process that funding agencies should take a strong-handed approach to upholding the expectations stipulated in the Minimum Standards in requests for proposals, grant evaluation, and review procedures and that indicators for measuring successful attainment of community engagement goals should align with the minimum standards.
- *Academic and research institutions:* As noted earlier, although advances in research regarding community-centered approaches are occurring, much work is still required to ensure standard measures are applied to the evaluation of community engagement approaches. In addition, there is limited research into how community engagement and associated approaches are seen through the lens of government planning, strategy, and budgeting, coordination across the humanitarian architecture at all levels, integration across work streams at all levels, and how resources are applied (e.g., making the business case for community engagement). Advancing a more nuanced research agenda informed by the Minimum Standards will provide much needed evidence toward greater accountability, prioritization, and impact.

Implications for the Overall Focus of the Book

Community engagement, as a concept and approach, has moved beyond discussions of the importance of participation and the establishment of feedback loops. The wide recognition of community engagement as a multidisciplinary approach requiring a supportive enabling environment has opened the conversation to include initiatives such as the Minimum Quality Standards and Indicators for Community

Engagement. These provide a framework for discussing, designing, delivering, measuring, and resourcing community engagement and supports in broadening the understanding of the role of all actors in a humanitarian response and their accountability to communities.

References

Abdullah, I., & Rashid, I. (2017). *Understanding west Africas Ebola epidemic: Towards a political economy*. Zed Books.

Abramowitz, S., McKune, S. L., Fallah, M., Monger, J., Tehoungue, K., & Omidian, P. A. (2017). The opposite of denial: Social learning at the onset of the Ebola emergency in Liberia. *Journal of Health Communication, 22*(Suppl 1), 59–65. https://doi.org/10.1080/10810730.2016.1209599

Abramowitz, S., McLean, K. E. E., McKune, S. L. L., et al. (2015). Community-centered responses to Ebola in urban Liberia: The view from below. *PLoS Neglected Tropical Diseases, 9*, e0003706.

Abramowitz, S., Rogers, B., Aklilu, L., Lee, S., & Hipgrave, D. (2016). *Ebola Community Care Centers: Lessons learned from UNICEF's 2014–2015 experience in Sierra Leone unite for children*. Retrieved December 16, 2017, from https://www.unicef.org/health/files/CCCReport_FINAL_July2016.pdf

Abramowitz, S. A., Hipgrave, D. B., Witchard, A., & Heymann, D. L. (2018). Lessons from the West Africa Ebola Epidemic: A systematic review of epidemiological and social and behavioral science research priorities. *The Journal of Infectious Diseases*. https://doi.org/10.1093/infdis/jiy387.

Ackerman Gulaid, L., & Kiragu, K. (2012). Lessons learnt from promising practices in community engagement for the elimination of new HIV infections in children by 2015 and keeping their mothers alive: Summary of a desk review. *Journal of the International AIDS Society, 15*(Suppl 2), 17390.

Alcayna-Stevens, L. (2018). *Planning for post-Ebola: Lessons learned from DR Congo's 9th epidemic*. Retrieved October 9, 2019, https://opendocs.ids.ac.uk/opendocs/handle/123456789/14450

Alpren, C., Jalloh, M. F., Kaiser, R., et al. (2017). The 117 call alert system in Sierra Leone: From rapid Ebola notification to routine death reporting. *BMJ Global Health, 2*, e000392.

Armstrong-Mensah, E. A., & Ndiaye, S. M. (2018). Global Health Security Agenda Implementation: A case for community engagement. *Health Security, 16*, 217–223.

Azad, K., Barnett, S., Banerjee, B., et al. (2010). Effect of scaling up women's groups on birth outcomes in three rural districts in Bangladesh: A cluster-randomised controlled trial. *Lancet, 375*, 1193–1202.

Baltzell, K., Harvard, K., Hanley, M., Gosling, R., & Chen, I. (2019). What is community engagement and how can it drive malaria elimination? Case studies and stakeholder interviews. *Malaria Journal, 18*, 245.

Bedford, J., Chitnis, K., Webber, N., Dixon, P., Limwame, K., Elessawi, R., & Obregon, R. (2017). Community engagement in Liberia: Routine immunization post-Ebola. *Journal of Health Communication, 22*(Suppl 1), 81–90. https://doi.org/10.1080/10810730.2016.1253122

Bedson, J., Jalloh, M. F., Pedi, D., et al. (2020). Community engagement during outbreak response: Standards, approaches, and lessons from the 2014-2016 Ebola outbreak in Sierra Leone. *BMJ Global Health, 5*, e002145.

Bedson, J., Skrip, L. A., Pedi, D., Abramowitz, S., et al. (2021). A review and agenda for integrated disease models including social andbehavioural factors. *Nature Human Behavior, 5*, 834–846. https://doi.org/10.1038/s41562-021-01136-2

Benton, A., & Dionne, K. Y. (2015). International political economy and the 2014 west African Ebola outbreak. *African Studies Review, 58*, 223–236.

Bonelli, F., Bourne, K., Broholm, E., et al. (2014). *Protection policy paper understanding community-based protection understanding community-based protection*. Retrieved April 18, 2018, from http://www.unhcr.org/ngo-consultations/ngo-consultations-2014/Understanding-Community-Based-Protection.pdf

Callis, A., Carter, V. M., Ramakrishnan, A., et al. (2018). Lessons learned in clinical trial communication during an Ebola outbreak: The implementation of STRIVE. *The Journal of Infectious Diseases, 217*, S40–S47.

Carter, S. E., Dietrich, L. M., & Minor, O. M. (2017). Mainstreaming gender in WASH: Lessons learned from Oxfam's experience of Ebola. *Gender and Development, 25*, 205–220.

Chandler, C., Fairhead, J., Kelly, A., et al. (2015). Ebola: Limitations of correcting misinformation. *Lancet, 385*, 1275–1277.

Dickmann, P., Kitua, A., Apfel, F., & Lightfoot, N. (2018). Kampala manifesto: Building community-based one health approaches to disease surveillance and response—The Ebola legacy—Lessons from a peer-led capacity-building initiative. *PLoS Neglected Tropical Diseases, 12*, e0006292.

Enria, L. (2019). The Ebola crisis in Sierra Leone: Mediating containment and engagement in humanitarian emergencies. *Development and Change, 50*(6), 1602–1623.

Enria, L., Lees, S., Smout, E., et al. (2016). Power, fairness and trust: Understanding and engaging with vaccine trial participants and communities in the setting up the EBOVAC-Salone vaccine trial in Sierra Leone. *BMC Public Health, 16*, 1140.

Frazer, A. (2019). *Post-Ebola case management of orphaned young adults in rural Sierra Leone*. Retrieved October 9, 2019, from https://scholarworks.waldenu.edu/cgi/viewcontent.cgi?article=7842&context=dissertations

Frieden, T. R. (2018). Still not ready for Ebola. *Science, 360*, 1049.

Gillespie, A. M., Obregon, R., El Asawi, R., et al. (2016). Social mobilization and community engagement central to the Ebola response in West Africa: Lessons for future public health emergencies. *Global Health: Science and Practice, 4*, 626–646.

Gilmore, B., Ndejjo, R., Tchetchia, A., et al. (2020). Community engagement for COVID-19 prevention and control: A rapid evidence synthesis. *BMJ Global Health, 5*, 3188.

Gray, N., Stringer, B., Bark, G., et al. (2018). 'When Ebola enters a home, a family, a community': A qualitative study of population perspectives on Ebola control measures in rural and urban areas of Sierra Leone. *PLoS Neglected Tropical Diseases, 12*, e0006461.

Groupe URD. (2009). *Participation handbook for humanitarian field workers*. Retrieved November 4, 2019, from https://www.urd.org/en/publication/participation-handbook-for-humanitarian-field-workers

Hansch, S., Sadaphal, S., Leigh, J., et al. (2018). *Evaluation of the USAID/OFDA Ebola virus disease outbreak response in West Africa 2014–2016*. Retrieved April 24, 2018, from https://pdf.usaid.gov/pdf_docs/PA00SSC3.pdf

Health Communications Capacity Collaborative. (2013). The process: Five steps to strategic communication. Retrieved May 3, 2018, from https://www.thehealthcompass.org/sites/default/files/strengthening_tools/ProcessEng%26Fr.pdf

Hewlett, B. S., & Amola, R. P. (2003). Cultural contexts of Ebola in northern Uganda. *Emerging Infectious Diseases, 9*, 1242–1248.

Hewlett, B. S., Epelboin, A., Hewlett, B. L., & Formenty, P. (2005). Medical anthropology and Ebola in Congo: Cultural models and humanistic care. *Bulletin de la Societe de Pathologie Exotique, 98*, 230–236.

Hewlett, B. S., & Hewlett, B. L. (2007). *Ebola, culture and politics: The anthropology of an emerging disease*. Cengage Learning.

Heymann, D. L. (2017). Ebola: Transforming fear into appropriate action. *Lancet, 390*, 219–220.

Heymann, D. L., Chen, L., Takemi, K., et al. (2015). Global health security: The wider lessons from the west African Ebola virus disease epidemic. *Lancet, 385*, 1884–1901.

Hoffman D. (2016). A Crouching village: Ebola and the empty gestures of quarantine in Monrovia. *City Society, 28*, 246–264.

Hofman, M., & Au, S. (2017). *The politics of fear: Médecins sans frontières and the west African Ebola epidemic*. Oxford University Press.

Houlihan, C. F., Youkee, D., & Brown, C. S. (2017). Novel surveillance methods for the control of Ebola virus disease. *International Health, 9*, 139–141.

Howard-Grabman, L., & Snetro, G. (2015). *How to mobilize communities for health and social change*. Retrieved April 19, 2018, from https://www.msh.org/sites/msh.org/files/2015_08_msh_how_to_mobilize_communities_for_health_social_change.pdf

Johnson, G., Bedford, J., McClelland, A., Tiffany, A., & Dalziel, B. (2015). *Evaluating the impact of safe and dignified burials for stopping Ebola transmission in West Africa—Summary findings from the anthropological study of Guinea*. Retrieved February 3, 2019, from www.anthrologica.com

Kangbai, J. B. (2016). Social network analysis and modeling of cellphone-based syndromic surveillance data for Ebola in Sierra Leone. *Asian Pacific Journal of Tropical Medicine, 9*(9), 851–855. https://doi.org/10.1016/j.apjtm.2016.07.005

Kateh, F., Nagbe, T., Kieta, A., et al. (2015). Rapid response to Ebola outbreaks in remote areas—Liberia, July-November 2014. *MMWR. Morbidity and Mortality Weekly Report, 64*, 188–192.

Larsen, T. M., Mburu, C. B., Kongelf, A., Tingberg, T., Sannoh, F., & Madar, A. A. (2017). Red Cross volunteers' experience with a mobile community event-based surveillance (CEBS) system in Sierra Leone during-and after the Ebola outbreak—A qualitative study. *Health and Primary Care*. doi: https://doi.org/10.15761/HPC.1000114.

Laverack, G., & Manoncourt, E. (2016). Key experiences of community engagement and social mobilization in the Ebola response. *Global Health Promotion, 23*(1), 79–82. https://doi.org/10.1177/1757975915606674

Lavery, J. V., Tinadana, P. O., Scott, T. W., et al. (2010). Towards a framework for community engagement in global health research. *Trends in Parasitology, 26*, 279–283.

Le Marcis, F. (2016). *Social immunization: Historical roots of population's response to the Ebola event in Guinea. Social sciences and biomedical engagements in the west African Ebola outbreak*. Institut Pasteur.

Le Marcis, F., Enria, L., Abramowitz, S., Saez, A., & Faye, S. L. B. (2019). Three acts of resistance during the 2014–16 West Africa Ebola epidemic. *Journal of Humanitarian Affairs*. https://doi.org/10.7227/JHA.014

Lee-Kwan, S. H., DeLuca, N., Adams, M., et al. (2014). Support services for survivors of Ebola virus disease-Sierra Leone, 2014. *Morbidity and Mortality Weekly Report, 63*, 1205–1206.

Lindblade, K. A., Kateh, F., Nagbe, T. K., et al. (2015). Decreased Ebola transmission after rapid response to outbreaks in remote areas, Liberia, 2014. *Emerging Infectious Diseases, 21*, 1800–1807.

Lipton, J. (2014). Care and burial practices in urban Sierra Leone. *Ebola Response Anthropology Platform*. Retrieved September 30, 2019, from http://www.ebola-anthropology.net/wp-content/uploads/2014/11/care-and-burial-practice.pdf

Mamadou Mbaye, E., Kone, S., Kâ, O., & Mboup, S. (2017). Évolution de l'implication des communautés dans la riposte à Ebola. *Sante Publique (Paris), 29*, 487.

Manguvo, A., & Mafuvadze, B. (2015). The impact of traditional and religious practices on the spread of Ebola in West Africa: Time for a strategic shift. *The Pan African Medical Journal, 22*(Suppl 1), 9.

Marston, C., Renedo, A., McGowan, C. R., & Portela, A. (2013). Effects of community participation on improving uptake of skilled care for maternal and newborn health: A systematic review. *PLoS One, 8*, e55012.

McCoy, D. C., Hall, J. A., & Ridge, M. (2012). A systematic review of the literature for evidence on health facility committees in low- and middle-income countries. *Health Policy and Planning, 27*(6), 449–466. https://doi.org/10.1093/heapol/czr077

McGovern, M. (2014). Bushmeat and the politics of disgust. *F Sites Hot Spots, Cult Anthropol Online*. Retrieved from https://culanth.org/fieldsights/bushmeat-and-the-politics-of-disgust

McMahon, S. A., Ho, L. S., Scott, K., et al. (2007). "We and the nurses are now working with one voice": How community leaders and health committee members describe their role in Sierra Leone's Ebola response. *BMC Health Services Research, 17*, 495.

McNeil, D. G., Jr. (2014). Outbreak in Sierra Leone is tied to single funeral where 14 women were infected. *New York Times, 163*, A7.

Medécins Sans Frontièrs. (2013). *Involving communities: Guidance document for approaching and cooperating with communities*. Retrieved August 12, 2019, from https://evaluation.msf.org/sites/evaluation/files/involving_communities_0.pdf

Mercy Corps. (2009). *Guide to community mobilization programming*. Retrieved April 17, 2018, from https://www.mercycorps.org/sites/default/files/CoMobProgrammingGd.pdf

Miller, N. P., Milsom, P., Johnson, G., et al. (2018). Community health workers during the Ebola outbreak in Guinea, Liberia, and Sierra Leone. *Journal of Global Health, 8*, 020601.

Milton, B., Attree, P., French, B., Povall, S., Whitehead, M., & Popay, J. (2012). The impact of community engagement on health and social outcomes: A systematic review. *Community Development Journal, 47*(3), 316–334. https://doi.org/10.1093/cdj/bsr043

Mobula, L. M., Nakao, J. H., Walia, S., Pendarvis, J., Morris, P., & Townes, D. (2018). A humanitarian response to the west African Ebola virus disease outbreak. *Journal of International Humanitarian Action, 3*, 10.

Moran, M. (2017). Missing bodies and secret funerals: The production of 'safe and dignified burials' in the Liberian Ebola crisis. *Anthropological Quarterly, 90*(2), 399–412.

Munodawafa, D., Moeti, M. R., Phori, P. M., et al. (2018). Monitoring and evaluating the Ebola response effort in two Liberian communities. *Journal of Community Health, 43*, 321–327.

Nagbe, T., Williams, G. S., Rude, J. M., et al. (2019). Lessons learned from detecting and responding to recurrent measles outbreak in Liberia post Ebola-epidemic 2016-2017. *The Pan African Medical Journal, 33*, 7.

Nau, J. Y. (2014). Ebola: Guide for burial and dignity. *Revue Médicale Suisse, 2014*(10), 2228–2229.

Nielsen, C. F., Kidd, S., Sillah, A. R. M., Davis, E., Mermin, J., & Kilmarx, P. H. (2015). Improving burial practices and cemetery management during an Ebola virus disease epidemic—Sierra Leone, 2014. *MMWR. Morbidity and Mortality Weekly Report, 64*, 20–27.

Nkangu, M. N., Olatunde, O. A., & Yaya, S. (2017). The perspective of gender on the Ebola virus using a risk management and population health framework: A scoping review. *Infectious Diseases of Poverty, 6*, 135.

Nyenswah, T., Massaquoi, M., Gbanya, M. Z., et al. (2015). Initiation of a ring approach to infection prevention and control at non-Ebola health care facilities—Liberia, January-February 2015. *MMWR. Morbidity and Mortality Weekly Report, 64*, 505–508.

Nyenswah, T. G., Kateh, F., Bawo, L., et al. (2016). Ebola and its control in Liberia, 2014-2015. *Emerging Infectious Diseases, 22*, 169–177.

Nyenswah, T. (2017). Reflections on leadership and governance from the incident manager of Liberia's Ebola response. *Health Security, 15*, 445–449.

OCHA. (2018). *Community engagement at the centre of disaster response*. Retrieved May 10, 2018, from https://www.unocha.org/story/community-engagement-centre-disaster-response

Odugleh-Kolev, A., & Parrish-Sprowl, J. (2018). Universal health coverage and community engagement. *Bulletin of the World Health Organization, 96*, 660–661.

Ottolenghi, E., Riveros, P., Blanding, S. (2018). *Assessment of the Bolivia Postabortion care community mobilization program the ACQUIRE project assessment of the Bolivia Postabortion care community mobilization program*. Retrieved December 13, 2018, from http://www.acquireproject.org/archive/files/5.0_community_engagement_marketing_and_communications/5.2_resources/5.2.2_studies/cPAC_report_revised_final.pdf

O'Mara-Eves, A., Brunton, G., Oliver, S., Kavanagh, J., Jamal, F., & Thomas, J. (2015). The effectiveness of community engagement in public health interventions for disadvantaged groups: A meta-analysis. *BMC Public Health, 15*, 129.

O'Sullivan, S., Sajid, M. I., Agusto, F. B., et al. (2018). Virtual autopsy and community engagement for outbreak response in Africa: Traditional, religious and sociocultural perspectives. *Egyptian Journal of Forensic Sciences., 8*, 67.

Parker, M., Hanson, T. M., Vandi, A., Sao Babawo, L., & Allen, T. (2019). Ebola, community engagement, and saving loved ones. *Lancet, 393*(10191), 2585. https://doi.org/10.1016/S0140-6736(19)31364-9

Pedi, D., Gillespie, A., Bedson, J., et al. (2017). The development of standard operating procedures for social mobilization and community engagement in Sierra Leone during the West Africa Ebola outbreak of 2014–2015. *Journal of Health Communication, 22*, 39–50.

Piot, P., Soka, M. J., & Spencer, J. (2019). Emergent threats: Lessons learnt from Ebola. *International Health, 11*, 334–337.

Popay, J., Attree, P., Hornby, D., et al. (2007). Community engagement in initiatives addressing the wider social determinants of health: A rapid review of evidence on impact, experience and process. *Social Determinanats Effectiveness Review*. Retrieved July 1, 2019, from Https://Www.Nice.Org.Uk/Guidance/Ph9/Documents/Social-Determinants-Evidence-Review-Final2

Quammen, D. (2014). *Ebola: The natural and human history of a deadly virus*. WW Norton & Company.

Ravi, S. J., Snyder, M. R., & Rivers, C. (2019). Review of international efforts to strengthen the global outbreak response system since the 2014–16 West Africa Ebola epidemic. *Health Policy and Planning, 34*, 47–54.

Richards, P., & Fairhead, J. (2014). Burial/other cultural practices and risk of EVD transmission in the Mano River Region. *Ebola Anthropology Response Platform*. Retrieved September 30, 2019, from http://www.ebola-anthropology.net/wp-content/uploads/2014/11/DFID-Brief-14oct14-burial-and-high-risk-cultural-practices-2.pdf

Richards, P. (2016). *Ebola: How a people's science helped end an epidemic*. Zed Books.

Richards, P., Amara, J., Mokuwa, E., Mokuwa, A., & Suluku, R. (2015a). *Village responses to Ebola virus disease in rural Central Sierra Leone—An interim report to the SMAC program, DFID Freetown. Ebola Response Anthropology Platform*. Njala University. Retrieved October 1, 2019, from http://www.ebola-anthropology.net/case_studies/village-responses-to-ebola-virus-disease-in-rural-central-sierra-leone/

Richards, P., Amara, J., Mokuwa, E., Mokuwa, A., & Suluku, R. (2015b). *Village responses to Ebola virus disease in rural eastern Sierra Leone—Second interim report to the SMAC program, DFID Freetown. Ebola Response Anthropology Platform*. Njala University. Retrieved October 1, 2019, from http://www.ebola-anthropology.net/case_studies/village-responses-to-ebola-virus-disease-in-rural-eastern-sierra-leone-second-interim-report/

Sacks, E., Swanson, R. C., Schensul, J. J., et al. (2017). Community involvement in health systems strengthening to improve Global Health Outcomes: A review of guidelines and potential roles. *International Quarterly of Community Health Education, 37*, 139–149.

Saez, A. M., & Borchert, M. (2014). Burial in times of Ebola—Dos and don't—Issues of acceptability. *Ebola Anthropology Response Platform*. Retrieved September 30, 2019, from http://www.ebola-anthropology.net/wp-content/uploads/2014/11/Burials-in-times-of-Ebola-Dos-and-donts-Acceptability-1.pdf

Schwartz, D. A., Anoko, J. N., & Abramowitz, S. A. (2019). *Pregnant in the time of Ebola: Women and their children in the 2013–2015 west African epidemic*. Springer.

Schwerdtle, P. M., De Clerck, V., & Plummer, V. (2017). Experiences of Ebola survivors: Causes of distress and sources of resilience. *Prehospital and Disaster Medicine, 32*(3), 234–239. https://doi.org/10.1017/S1049023X17000073. Epub 2017 Feb 20. PMID: 28215187.

Sepers, C. E., Fawcett, S. B., Hassaballa, I., et al. (2019). Evaluating implementation of the Ebola response in Margibi County, Liberia. *Health Promotion International, 34*, 510–518.

Shultz, J. M., Cooper, J. L., Baingana, F., et al. (2016). The role of fear-related behaviors in the 2013-2016 West Africa Ebola virus disease outbreak. *Current Psychiatry Reports, 18*, 104.

Social Mobilisation Action Consortium. (2014). Community-Led Ebola Action (CLEA) field guide for community mobilisers. Freetown, Sierra Leone. Retrieved April 17, 2018, from http://www.communityledtotalsanitation.org/blog/community-led-ebola-action-adapting-community-led-approach-ebola-outbreak-sierra-leone

Storey, J. D., Chitnis, K., Obregon, R., & Garrison, K. (2017). Community engagement and the communication response to Ebola. *Journal of Health Communication, 22*, 2–4.

Tambo, E., Chengho, C. F., Ugwu, C. E., Wurie, I., Jonhson, J. K., & Ngogang, J. Y. (2017). Rebuilding transformation strategies in post-Ebola epidemics in Africa. *Infectious Diseases of Poverty, 6*, 71.

Tedrow, V. A., Zelaya, C. E., Kennedy, C. E., et al. (2012). No "'magic bullet'": Exploring community mobilization strategies used in a multi-site community based randomized controlled trial: Project accept (HPTN 043). https://doi.org/10.1007/s10461-011-0009-9

Tindana, P. O., Singh, J. A., Tracy, C. S., et al. (2007). Grand challenges in global health: Community engagement in research in developing countries. *PLoS Medicine, 2007*(4), e273.

Tripathy, P., Nair, N., Barnett, S., et al. (2010). Effect of a participatory intervention with women's groups on birth outcomes and maternal depression in Jharkhand and Orissa, India: A cluster-randomised controlled trial. *Lancet, 375*, 1182–1192.

UNDP United Nations Development Programme. (2016). Sustainable development goals. Sdg7. https://doi.org/10.1017/CBO9781107415324.004

United Nations Children's Fund (UNICEF). (2020). Minimum quality standards and indicators for community engagement, New York.

United Nations High Commission on Refugees (UNHCR). (2008). *A community-based approach in UNHCR operations*. Retrieved April 20, 2018, from http://www.refworld.org/pdfid/47da54722.pdf

Victora, C. G., & Barros, F. C. (2013). Participatory women's groups: Ready for prime time? *Lancet, 381*, 1693–1694.

Wallerstein, N., & Duran, B. (2010). Community-based participatory research contributions to intervention research: The intersection of science and practice to improve health equity. *American Journal of Public Health, 100*(Suppl 1), S40–S46. https://doi.org/10.2105/AJPH.2009.184036

Walsh, S., & Johnson, O. (2018). *Getting to zero: A doctor and a diplomat on the Ebola Frontline*. Zed Books.

Wilkinson, A., Lipton, J., Martineau, F., & Chandler, C. (2014). Mobilising informal health workers for the Ebola response: Potential and programme considerations—Briefing note. *Ebola Anthropology Response Platform*. Retrieved November 14, 2019, from http://www.ebola--anthropology.net/wp-content/uploads/2014/11/Mobilising-informal-health-workers-Ebola-Response-Anthropology-Platform.pdf

Wilkinson, A., Parker, M., Martineau, F., & Leach, M. (2017). Engaging 'communities': Anthropological insights from the west African Ebola epidemic. *Philosophical Transactions of the Royal Society Series B, Biological Sciences, 372*(1721), 20160305. https://doi.org/10.1098/rstb.2016.0305

World Health Assembly. (2005). *International health regulations*. Retrieved November 5, 2020, from https://www.who.int/publications/i/item/9789241580496

World Health Organization (WHO). (2020). *COVID-19 global risk communication and community engagement strategy*. Retrieved June 8, 2021, from https://www.rcce-collective.net/resource/covid-19_rcce_globalstrategy2020/

Part II
Case Studies: Learning from Practice

Chapter 4
Reflections on Social Behavior Change: Lessons Learned from Polio Outbreak Response

Sahar Hegazi and Sam Oumo Okiror

Contents

Background

Since 1988, when the World Health Assembly (WHA) challenged the World Health Organization (WHO) to coordinate the eradication of wild polioviruses worldwide, five organizations—WHO, Rotary International (RI), UNICEF, the Bill and Melinda Gates Foundation (BMGF), and the US Centers for Disease Control and Prevention (CDC)—have spearheaded the initiative to eradicate polio and was recently joined by Global Alliance for Vaccination Initiative (GAVI). Over the past 32 years, the initiative has made extraordinary progress. Wild poliovirus cases have dropped from an estimated 350,000 cases a year in 1988 to only 140 wild polioviruses type 1 as of December 31, 2020 (GPEI, 2020). Endemic transmission has continued in only two countries, Afghanistan and Pakistan, but currently, circulating vaccine-deprived polio virus (cVDPV) outbreaks pose new challenges to the overall mission

S. Hegazi (✉)
UNICEF Regional Office for South Asia (ROSA), Amman, Jordan
e-mail: shegazi@unicef.org

S. O. Okiror
Rapid Response Team/WHO Africa Region Office (AFRO), Brazzaville, Congo

E. Manoncourt et al. (eds.), *Communication and Community Engagement in Disease Outbreaks*, https://doi.org/10.1007/978-3-030-92296-2_4

to eradicate polio with 918 cases of cVDPV reported in 25 countries worldwide by end of December 2020.

Nigeria was removed from the list of endemic countries as of August 2020 after at least 3 years without confirmed wild poliovirus in the presence of certification level surveillance—resulting in the African Region becoming the fifth WHO region to be certified wild poliovirus-free, joining The Americas, Western Pacific, European and South East Asia Regions, with only the Eastern Mediterranean remaining polio endemic. Areas with continuing polio transmission have some common characteristics. These are areas with low routine immunization in general but specifically for polio, are hard to reach attributable to geographical and/or security challenges, have high numbers of mobile population, or acceptance of vaccine is low with vaccination not perceived as a child health priority among those communities. Meanwhile, the emergence of circulating vaccine-derived polio virus type 2 in particular (cVDPV2) has further complicated the communication task where demand for vaccination should be maintained above 90% among communities with virus circulation and refusals should be less than 1% among families with children under 5 years of age (SOPs Version 3 Jan 2019).

The COVID-19 pandemic has had a deleterious effect on the polio eradication efforts. All outbreak response campaigns were stopped, active surveillance for paralyzed children was significantly compromised as countries implemented total lockdowns. Again, communication was viewed as a key enabler for the resumption of polio campaigns in a context that pushed polio low on the public agenda of interest. The global polio Standard Operating Procedures (SOPs) provide five important elements to a successful response to a polio outbreak. First, there is a need to have fully engaged national and subnational governments; second, rapid detection, notification investigation, and risk assessment; third, a strong advocacy, communication, and social mobilization; fourth, a robust immunization response; and last, a high-quality and enhanced surveillance system. The role played by a robust advocacy, communication, and social mobilization in facilitating all the major elements of outbreak response cannot be overemphasized. Unless Communication for Development (C4D) is at the forefront of generating demand for immunization and obtaining community acceptance for vaccine and building community commitment to vaccination as an important health practice, refusals for polio vaccination cannot be minimized. Failure to accelerate this component of the SOPs could risk delaying interrupting transmission requiring more resources, and seed community fatigue due to many repeated campaigns.

It is critical to conduct political advocacy to enlist support for polio eradication in the face of other emergencies and public health priorities that governments have to balance against a disappearing disease, albeit because of the successes achieved over the years. Invariably, at the highest political level, acceptance may be secured but how this trickles down to the community and translates to reaching over 90% of children with viable vaccine hinges a lot on community mobilization at the operational level to enlist their full participation and empowerment. The complexities of effectively realizing this work at the community level depend on several factors, including understanding the social and cultural norms, religious inclinations, and communication channels, to mention but a few. As such, as outlined in Chap. 1, social and behavioral factors must be woven into the overarching global architecture of disease outbreak, as well as preparedness and response for such public health emergencies.

The subsequent sections outline some of the communication approaches employed in the polio outbreak response using case studies and drawing some key lessons for future health communication interventions targeting disease outbreaks.

Communication Approaches

The global polio eradication SOPs, Version 3 Jan 2019, consider communication as a key component in an outbreak response that would: (a) strengthen all response activities' performance, (b) increase uptake of vaccination among target population groups, and (c) support robust surveillance with early notification of acute flaccid paralysis (AFP) cases. However, in the context of vaccine-derived poliovirus, communicating risk and ensuring demand during vaccination campaigns could be a challenging mission to achieve, particularly for countries that: (1) have not seen polio cases for years, (2) stopped using OPV, or (3) when the virus is detected only in the environment and/or only a limited number of cases are reported. In the context of the outbreak response, the SOPs outline the role of communication in raising awareness of campaign dates, strengthening community perceptions of vaccination by building trust in health worker capacity in vaccine safety and efficacy, and elevating the perception of polio risk, which would contribute to high coverage of the targeted children. These factors are reflected in the UNICEF model for the decision to vaccinate.

Since the withdrawal of the trivalent oral polio vaccine (tOPV) vaccine in 2016 and with the increased number of countries responding to polio outbreaks due to a drop in population immunity, particularly against polio virus type 2, only a few countries were able to interrupt the virus transmission within the recommended 120 days.

By reviewing outbreak countries' plans and final assessment reports at the closure of the outbreaks over the last 4 years, we found several common factors that could have positively influenced maintaining high public demand for vaccination such as: (a) effective partnerships especially between UNICEF and WHO; (b) availability of an in-country team to undertake the communication planning and response as soon as the outbreak is confirmed; and (c) availability of implementing agencies with acceptable capacity, and expertise and resources.

From a communication perspective, the key enabling factors included the availability of trusted and functioning community engagement networks; public access to communication channels such as mass media or social media, and availability of timely social data to: (a) guide program planning and implementation and (b) measure the effectiveness of strategies under implementation and suggest required amendments. However, none of this would have been fully effective without government leadership and commitment to outbreak response activities particularly by reaching targeted children, especially among the hard-to-reach populations.

With the guidance of UNICEF, most countries responding to outbreaks adopted a similar communication model mainly dependent on information sharing and education. In situations where a full community engagement model was planned and implemented, the results exceeded the outbreak response goals and were sustained beyond closure of the outbreak to benefit boosting demand for routine immunization. Taking an example such as Ukraine mentioned in the next section, the communication strategies were tactfully planned to ensure informing and working with communities but also to empower them to engage and express their concerns, if any. This was envisaged as an important process especially after an earlier incident of death of a child following measles vaccine leading to widespread anti-vaccine sentiments. This comprehensive approach helped to create demand for vaccination beyond the polio outbreak which was sustained for years after. In most of those cases, countries' communication outbreak response plans were characterized by using a blended communication approach where information, education, and communication (IEC) was only one of several tools rather than the main strategy. This is confirmed by Weiss et al., who suggested that while IEC activities helped increase access to routine immunizations, IEC activities do not appear sufficient to achieve high levels of routine immunization coverage. Longer-term relationships between caretakers and local health workers who support childhood immunizations appear more important and may reflect issues of trust in the health system.

Strategies that promote immunization also need to be tailored to the religious and educational background of families and caretakers. Countries such as Ethiopia, Kenya, and South Sudan that planned and implemented systematic community engagement as part of their outbreak response effort were able to maintain refusals below 1% had at least one or more of the following elements. First, community engagement interventions were done through mobilizers recruited from the same community and trained in health communications and interpersonal communications techniques. Second, community leaders, health professionals, and other influencers were engaged in the pre-campaign planning to support and publicly promote the importance of vaccinations among their constituencies and finally understand and address any concerns in between campaigns. This conclusion was indicated by Curry et al., who demonstrated caregivers who reported a visit by community mobilizers were more likely to fully immunize their children against polio. In Ethiopia and India, caregivers who recalled a visit by the community mobilizer were significantly and positively associated with routine polio vaccination completion.

On the other hand, mass and social media are also effective platforms for reaching caretakers, especially for a widely dispersed population or in countries with high media coverage and fewer community networks. Several studies highlight the influence of media on reaching positive results of mass campaigns. For example, Weiss et al. indicated that after a mass campaign in Pakistan, missed children were more likely to have lived in homes without a TV or a radio or have a caretaker who reported not being informed at least 1 day in advance of the campaign. It was also reported in the same study that in Egypt, children who missed polio campaigns were more likely to have a caretaker who did not watch TV or who reported having a limited number of information sources.

Reaching the hard-to-reach through communication outbreak response activities is critical to support the operational and epidemiological efforts to contain an outbreak. In some countries, minority ethnic or religious groups are usually associated with lower vaccination rates, especially during vaccination campaigns. For example, in India, Muslims were the last religious group where polio virus circulation continued until the country successfully eradicated the disease. This was attributed mistrust of minorities about the intentions of their national government and health providers leading to their refusal of the services provided. In other instances, health providers may neglect to prioritize the services to minorities, for example, remote clinics in areas of Pashtun communities in Pakistan and in the slums of Karachi did not have regular medical services, since those communities are not prioritized by their governments.

In the next section, we would like to present two case studies for two countries that managed to interrupt virus circulation and close the outbreak in a time-bound period of within 120 days as recommended in the SOPs despite numerous challenges faced.

The first example is Ukraine, which eradicated polio in early 2000 as part of the WHO European Region (WHO/EURO) certification as polio-free. However, in late 2015, two vaccine-derived polio virus type 1 were confirmed in one district in the southwest of the country. At that time, Ukraine's overall routine immunization rate was estimated to be around 17%, and inactivated polio vaccine (IPV) was the only vaccine used in the country. Additionally, the health authorities did not approve of mass campaigns and insisted on organizing the response to focus on inviting caretakers to go to health clinics.

The second example to be presented is from Syria, a country under civil war for more than 8 years. A type 2 vaccine-derived polio virus outbreak was confirmed in one of the districts in the eastern part of the country in an area controlled by ISIS. Due to the low immunity of children in those areas and elsewhere in the country, more than 70 children were paralyzed as a result of the outbreak. Organizing mass campaigns in this region was quite complex as it had to be coordinated with both the national government and ISIS to allow the vaccination campaigns to take place. The outbreak's spread to other areas that were under Kurdish authorities introducing other layers of negotiations and complications.

Ukraine Unique Challenge: Responding to an Outbreak in Low Immunization Environment

On August 28, 2015, the Polio Regional Reference Laboratory in Moscow notified the WHO Regional Office for Europe that two cases of circulating vaccine-derived poliovirus type 1 (cVDPV1) had been discovered in the Zakarpatiya region of southwest Ukraine. The following day, WHO alerted the Global Polio Eradication Initiative (GPEI) partnership about these two children—a 4-year-old boy and 10-month-old girl—and on September 1, the Ukrainian Minister of Health made a public announcement of the outbreak. GPEI Standard Operating Procedures for response to a polio outbreak, as well as its Polio Communications Global Toolkit, formed the blueprint for the response. International agencies, particularly UNICEF and WHO, mobilized instantly to provide daily advice to the Ukrainian health ministry. UNICEF assisted the ministry with the development of a crisis communication plan to immediately respond to the outbreak. Coordinating and advisory bodies were established immediately, in keeping with SOPs. A parallel communications task force, spearheaded by UNICEF, activated its pre-positioned outbreak response plan. Implementation of the response, however, never enjoyed whole-of-government support. Additionally, a national public health emergency was never declared, which does not conform with the World Health Assembly (WHA)-established standards.

Ukraine's history of vaccine hesitancy and refusal highlights the enormity of the communication challenge. Both caregivers and, in some cases, health professionals lacked trust in vaccines. The first major communication challenge was addressing the widespread denial that there was an outbreak at all. The national government did not adequately communicate news of the outbreak to regional and district authorities, which signaled a relaxed approach to the outbreak response. This had a cascading effect on the initial communication plan, hence the public communication tone.

Unprecedented challenges existed even before the polio outbreak occurred. In 2008, a child died after measles vaccination. The anti-vaccinator lobby, which has a strong ground in Ukraine, used this incident to destroy the program's reputation. The negative impact of this incident has lasted for years. Thus, when the outbreak was confirmed, pharmaceutical importers were spearheading not only aggressive opposition to rational purchase of vaccines but supported anti-vaccine media coverage. Meanwhile, professional health workers were often confused, telling parents different stories in public and in private. The medical community was divided with some physicians being supporters while others were opponents of vaccination. For example, some pediatricians would often advise caretakers against immunization for fear of side effects.

The planned three rounds of vaccination campaigns to contain the virus circulation encountered a number of roadblocks. Anti-vaccine rumors continued to circulate in the media, especially social media. However, the well-planned and implemented communication for behavior and social change interventions promoted public acceptance, and demand was reinforced. This contributed to significant increase in vaccine coverage from below 17% (3 polio doses in children under 1 year of age) in 2015 before the outbreak to 65% in Round 1 and 75% in Round 2 (targeting age 2 months to 6 years), and 82% in Round 3 (targeting age 10 months to 10 years). While falling below the 95% international standard, these results were significant within Ukraine's unique and challenging context.

The communication response involved: adherence to GPEI guidelines, application of the polio communication global toolkit, and employment of best practices for handling polio outbreaks, taking full advantage of local knowledge and available opportunities. Many of the elements of the immediate response communication phase were already in place at the time of the outbreak, including analysis of the media landscape and creation of straightforward announcement messages, intended to maximize awareness of the outbreak and impending vaccine campaigns. The premise underlying the C4D strategy was imperative to overcome vaccine hesitancy—derived from an array of factors including denial of the outbreak, fear of adverse consequences of vaccination, and lack of trust in the source of the vaccines—among two key populations: parents/caregivers and health workers. The communication interventions also emerged into three phases and after each vaccination round were readapted as ongoing research uncovered specific fears, rumors, and other new issues. As a result, images, tone, and messages for the public communication and media campaign changed to a more specific and bold approach that utilized the fear appeal. They capitalized on the fact that Ukraine public is educated and has almost universal access to television, the internet, and social media. In line with that finding, the theory of change and assumptions included in the outbreak response communication plan were reviewed. The images and messages moved from a simplistic approach aiming at creating just awareness to a fully rounded approach that considers different behavior models such as social learning and social norms as shown in Fig. 4.1.

Three rounds of public polls were undertaken immediately after each vaccination campaign through patient exist interviews and in crowded public places using polio global monitoring tools. The sample was representative of total Ukraine as well as urban and rural populations from different geographical zones of the country. Overall, the communication interventions created quite a high awareness or polio disease (96% for third vaccination round), which was statistically significant when compared with data collected after the first poll (89%) as noted in Fig. 4.2.

The same figure was only 68% in 2014 when the same question was asked as part of a national knowledge, attitudes, and practice (KAP) undertaken before the outbreak. Additionally, after the first round public knowledge of the response to the outbreak was 58%, this improved to 66% after Round 2 and 70% after Round 3 of the campaigns.

Overall, the communication interventions contributed to reducing reasons for missed children from the first to third round except for some reasons for refusals as shown in Fig. 4.3.

Correlation between exposure to polio messages through mass media and refusals showed a statistically significant reduction when data for rounds 1 and 3 were compared, as shown in Fig. 4.4.

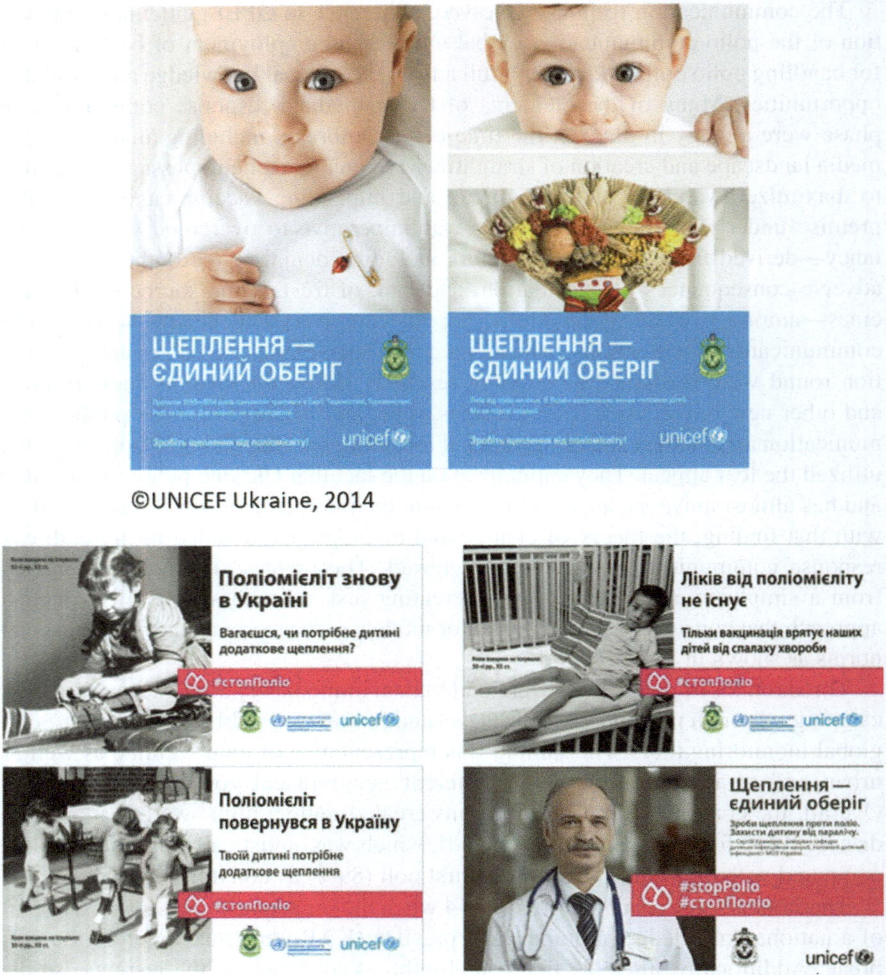
ЩЕПЛЕННЯ —
ЄДИНИЙ ОБЕРІГ
Зробіть щеплення від поліомієліту!
unicef
ЩЕПЛЕННЯ —
ЄДИНИЙ ОБЕРІГ
unicef
©UNICEF Ukraine, 2014
Поліомієліт знову в Україні
Вагаєшся, чи потрібне дитині додаткове щеплення?
#стопПоліо
unicef
Ліків від поліомієліту не існує
Тільки вакцинація врятує наших дітей від спалаху хвороби
#стопПоліо
unicef
Поліомієліт повернувся в Україну
Твоїй дитині потрібне додаткове щеплення
#стопПоліо
unicef
Щеплення — єдиний оберіг
Зроби щеплення проти поліо.
Захисти дитину від паралічу.
#stopPolio
#стопПоліо
unicef
©UNICEF Ukraine, 2015

Fig. 4.1 Public communication images before Round 1 and adapted after Round 1

On the other hand, the correlation between exposure to polio messages through health providers and refusals showed an increase in refusals between Rounds 1 and 3 for those caretakers citing health providers as their prime source of information, which implies a negative role played by health providers. The top reasons mentioned for refusal include the vaccine not being safe and fear of side effects, especially among those most exposed to relevant polio messages through their health providers. Those results led to refocusing the communication interventions in the following 6 months after the outbreak to be entirely targeting health providers and private practitioners, especially in remote areas and among resisting groups.

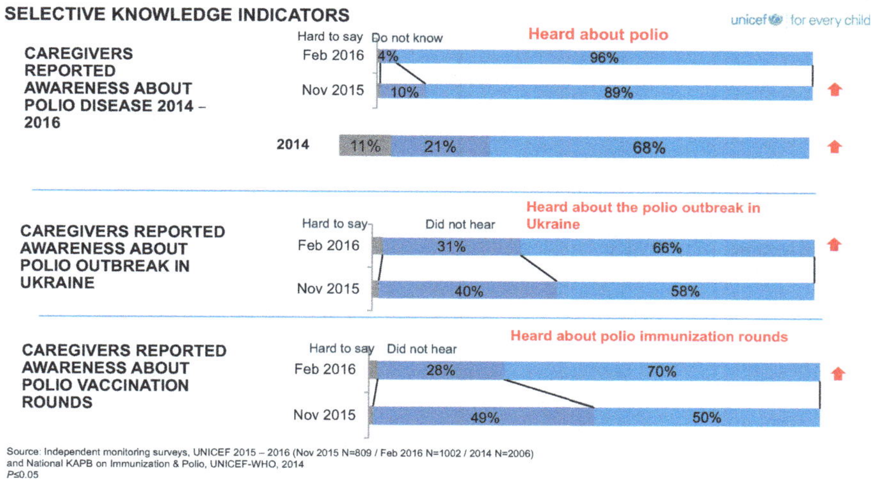

Fig. 4.2 Selective knowledge indicators

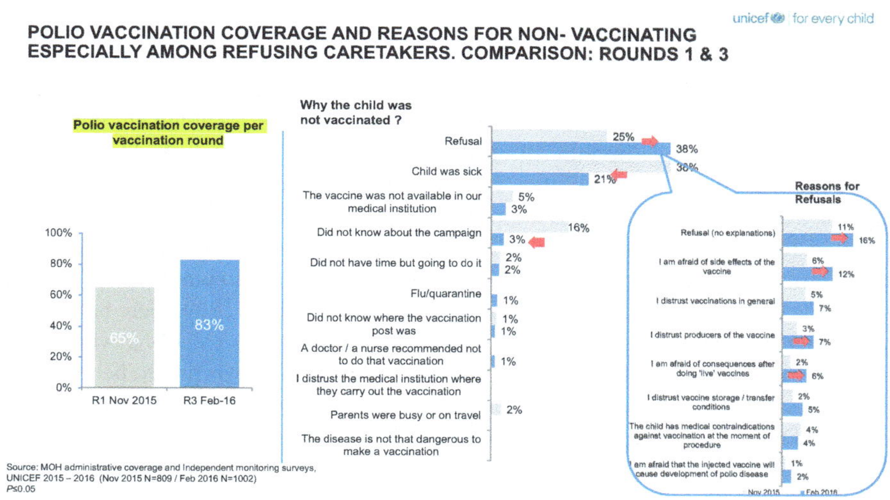

Fig. 4.3 Polio vaccination coverage and reasons for non-vaccinating especially among refusing caretakers. Comparison: Rounds 1 and 3

Syria: Responding to an Outbreak in a War Zone

On June 2, 2017, the Syrian Ministry of Health confirmed a second case of circulating vaccine-derived polio virus type 2 (cVDPV2) in an area of Deir-ez-Zor governorate controlled by the Islamic State (ISIS), signaling a polio outbreak and setting in motion an outbreak response, consisting of several vaccination rounds for

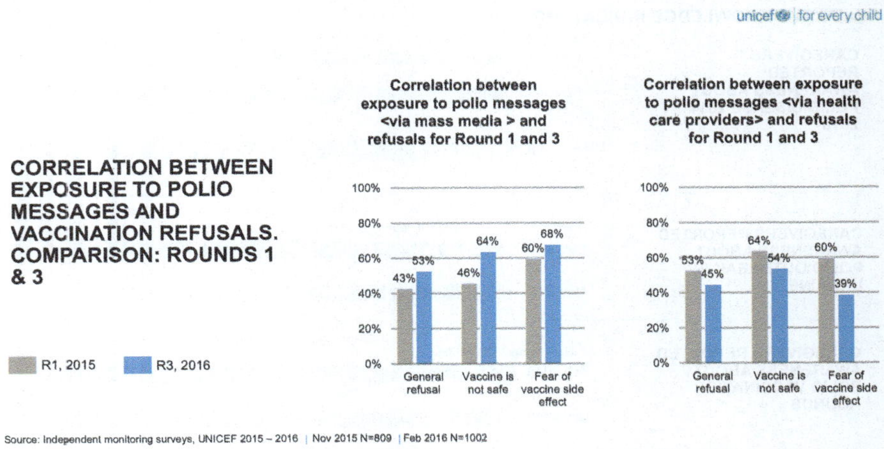

Fig. 4.4 Correlation between exposure to polio messages and vaccination refusals. Comparison: Rounds 1 and 3

children under the age of 5 years. The same area had experienced a wild polio outbreak a few years earlier (2013–2014), which took more than 8 months to halt, due in part to UN agencies' inability to operate in areas controlled by ISIS or other opposition groups [ref]. A series of 13 national vaccination campaigns took place from 2013 to 2016, including multi-antigen campaigns that provided all childhood vaccination to improve immunization coverage that had dramatically deteriorated since the start of the Syrian conflict. However, the multi-antigen campaigns in Deir-ez-Zor were not completed due to opposition from ISIS, and coverage was low (e.g., 49% in Round 2) [MAIC report]. This resulted in an immunity gap in the local population in this governorate, making it ripe for another polio outbreak.

While type 2 wild polio virus was eradicated worldwide in 1999, there have been a number of outbreaks of type 2 vaccine-derived polio virus (VDPV), which can occur when the vaccine virus mutates over time, eventually reverting to be virulent, infecting, and paralyzing children in areas with low polio vaccination coverage, such as Deir-ez-Zor. As with other polio outbreaks, it requires a rapid response in the form of two or more rounds of vaccination campaigns for all children under 5 years in the affected areas (GPEI SOPs). The 2017 outbreak resulted in 74 cases—all infected children were from Deir-ez-Zor, except for 2 from Rikka, making it one of the largest circulating vaccine-derived polio virus type 2 (cVDPV2) outbreaks ever reported. The outbreak was met with a robust response, consisting of three rounds of the monovalent oral polio vaccine type 2 (mOPV2) and one round of inactivated polio vaccine (IPV). This response took place under extremely challenging conditions, including an active conflict with frequent airstrikes, divided control of the target governorates by different factions involved in the conflict, distrust of the local population towards the local or national authorities, the destruction of health facilities, mass media infrastructure and mass population movements as the conflict intensified.

A critical element of the response was the C4D activities to overcome the population's mistrust of the vaccine and possible resistance to the vaccination campaigns. Frequent airstrikes, lack of electricity and other basic services, and the disruption of mass communications, combined with the fluid political situation, led to high levels of mistrust of the local residents in Deir-ez-Zor toward the public health services and the idea of vaccination teams making home visits. This presented a further challenge to the communication effort and overall outbreak response. After a VDPV case was detected in Raqqa, it was decided to extend the vaccination campaigns to this governorate, where the situation was quite different. Kurdish forces had already taken control of much of the governorate from ISIS. Much of the population had fled to internally displaced persons (IDP) camps, where the vaccination campaigns largely took place.

Once the Ministry of Health (MOH) confirmed the outbreak, the WHO focal point working in Deir-ez-Zor began the task of establishing a network of community mobilizers who are young people residing in the areas to be targeted, and this network became the backbone of the communications and social mobilization activities during the response. These volunteers included current and former health workers, university students idled by the closure of schools, traditional birth attendants, and other community members who were recruited in consultation with local authorities and community leaders, such as tribal leaders, mayors (Mokhtars), and village chiefs.

The community mobilizers were responsible for making home visits prior to the vaccination campaigns, where possible, to distribute educational materials to inform residents about the campaign dates, urge caretakers to immunize their children during the campaign, and to identify potential cases of hesitancy or refusals to be addressed. In addition, community meetings were organized by some of the natural and religious leaders to reassure families regarding the vaccination teams and the importance of seizing this vaccination opportunity to protect the children and the entire community.

Support from influential community members, especially private physicians, was sought to address concerns of families regarding vaccine safety and any other related issue. Other community leaders such as heads of schools and/or respected teachers conducted some home visits to follow up with families refusing vaccination or whose children were missed in the campaign. Community mobilizers were trained through a cascading approach. A small group received training using materials developed by UNICEF in Damascus that covered interpersonal communications techniques (through roleplaying), key messages to convey, strategies for managing vaccine refusal, and community engagement techniques.

The community mobilizers were organized in teams of 20, each headed by a team leader. A total of 540 community mobilizers took part in the outbreak response in Deir-ez-Zor and Raqqa during both phases combined, with coverage of at least one volunteer in every community in the target areas. While they received some compensation for meals and transportation—but no salaries—a key motivating factor for these volunteers was the opportunity to be useful to their communities that felt marginalized and lacked public health services.

Given the political and social conditions under which the population in Deir-ez-Zor was living, as well as a history of vaccine refusal in the governorate, it was decided to conduct a rapid household survey in areas of expected response to determine the level of community acceptance or resistance to the upcoming polio vaccination campaigns and identify potential social barriers to and misconceptions about the vaccination to inform the development of key messages. The survey was conducted over a 2-week period by 300 social mobilizers and other volunteers and made possible by delays in the vaccination campaign, and consisted of a purposive sample of 6969 caregivers who were interviewed, using a brief questionnaire, about their intent to have their children vaccinated, reasons for refusing vaccination, perceived attitudes toward vaccines in the community, and their trusted sources of information. The data were entered and analyzed by a locally hired team of data analysts in Deir-ez-Zor.

The survey identified areas of resistance to the polio vaccination campaigns—often entire streets—and found that overall, 32% of caregivers (2242 out of 6969) would refuse to have their children vaccinated, with many citing concerns or rumors about the vaccine's source, safety, or effectiveness; the fact that their children were already vaccinated; and advice from their pediatricians against vaccination (especially IPV) were among the reasons for refusal. The survey also identified influential community members, including Mokhtars, mothers-in-law, and health workers, as their main trusted sources of information.

The results of this rapid survey, supplemented by data from Deir-ez-Zor from a 2016 knowledge, attitudes, and practice (KAP) survey on the population's knowledge and perceptions about polio vaccination and information sources, were used to fine-tune the specific communications activities and craft the main messages to counter the misperceptions and arguments against polio vaccination found in the survey. These activities and messages were incorporated into the C4D plan and activities.

Community mobilizers conducted a "social mapping" exercise in each community to identify individuals who could positively or negatively influence the community's views toward the polio vaccination campaign. These included religious leaders (e.g., Imams of mosques), tribal chiefs, teachers, pediatricians, and other doctors, female elders, traditional birth attendants, IDP camp managers (in Raqqa only), and local government council staff. The team lead of each community mobilizers' group met with these "influencers" individually or in groups to sensitize them about the campaign and communicated key messages to refute vaccine refusals in order to secure their support for the campaigns and even their active participation in promoting them and in reducing vaccine resistance within their communities. This included visits to hundreds of private pediatricians prior to the campaigns to help address vaccine hesitancy. Eighty-five of these community leaders and influencers in Deir-ez-Zor and Raqqa also took part in formal C4D training prior to Round 1.

A critical part of this effort prior to and during the campaigns was to persuade community influencers who were resistant to or actively preaching against polio vaccination—such as the tribal chief in a village that experienced many deaths at the hands of ISIS and was therefore mistrustful of a campaign that had its support, the influential grandmother urging 46 of her female neighbors not to have their children vaccinated, and the private physicians wary of the vaccine—to support the campaign. There is anecdotal evidence that these influencers played a key role in addressing the issue of trust in the vaccine and the vaccination team in Deir-ez-Zor and convincing people to have their children vaccinated over multiple rounds.

Given the high rate of refusals found in the initial pre-vaccination survey in Deir-ez-Zor, the C4D activities' primary focus was to address the issue of vaccine hesitancy before the campaign began instead of waiting to see who missed vaccination once the campaign was underway. This allowed more time for the C4D teams to try to reverse these refusals. To meet this objective, the UNICEF C4D team developed a refusal tracking system. Five to 7 days before each vaccination round, the community mobilizers would visit each household with children under five in their assigned area (where permitted by local authorities) to inform them about the campaign date and to identify potential refusal cases. A refusal card was completed for each resistant household, which included information on the reasons for refusal, where they obtained the information or advice against vaccination, and who they trusted and were influenced by.

The data from these cards were summarized by team leaders in a daily report, which included recommendations for adjusting community activities based on the findings and rumors in the community. The data were also entered daily onto a refusal tracking spreadsheet, which listed each resistant household, reason for refusal, the proposed strategy for follow-up for each case, and whether or not the children were eventually vaccinated ("resolved refusal case"). This information was also visualized on a dashboard prepared at the UNICEF regional office in Amman, Jordan during Phase 1, making it easier to readily identify resistant areas and the progress in resolving cases.

All reported refusal cases were followed up through home visits by a community mobilizer and one or more community influencers. Which influencer(s) to send and what messages to convey were determined by the caregiver's responses. If, for instance, he or she cited concerns about the vaccine's source or safety, a pediatrician or other health worker would take part in the follow-up home visit. In contrast, an objection to vaccination on religious grounds would result in a visit by a religious leader.

Other community communication channels, in addition to household visits, were used to reach as many people as possible with information about the campaigns in a short timeframe. For example, especially in areas or during periods where home visits were not possible, small group meetings became a major communication forum to convey information about the disease or address any community concern regarding the vaccine and the campaigns. These included meetings led by community and religious leaders targeting fathers as well as awareness sessions for mothers and grandmothers. With approval from local authorities, 350 mosques in

Deir-ez-Zor and Raqqa were used to make campaign announcements over loud-speakers and during Friday prayers during Phase 1 of the outbreak response. Public service announcements and scripted interviews with local doctors were broadcast on locally run radio stations in both the governorates. At the same time, announcements were also made by community mobilizers using megaphones in vehicles that traveled through the different communities, especially the remote ones in the desert. Educational materials were distributed at multiple venues and through different channels to maximize their reach. These included banners placed at village entrances or other highly visible areas. As a reminder, prior to each campaign, more than 30,000 campaign date inserts were added into bread bags at participating bakeries in Deir-ez-Zor, and posters with key messages were placed on water distribution trucks and fixed water tanks, which the population was heavily dependent on for drinking water. In all, more than 500,000 printed IEC materials, including leaflets, posters, and banners, were distributed to households, pharmacists, shops, doctors' offices, and other venues during both the phases of the response. As a further incentive to vaccinate, given the lack of clean water in the area, the C4D teams distributed vouchers to families in Deir-ez-Zor, enabling them to receive bottles of AquaTabs once their children were vaccinated. This disinfectant was also widely distributed during the campaigns in Raqqa, with the assistance of the community mobilizers, to ensure their proper distribution and safe use.

During and immediately following the campaigns, C4D teams worked with the vaccination teams to identify households with children who had not been vaccinated. Using tally sheets, they would conduct follow-up visits to determine the reason. Refusal cases would receive additional visits by community influencers and community mobilizers. For those who agreed to have their children vaccinated, as well as children who were unvaccinated for other reasons, such as illness or being missed by the vaccination team, vaccinators made follow-up visits during the campaign or mop-up period or requested the families to visit a health facility where the vaccine was available.

Following each round, data from independent monitoring (IM) surveys on the public's knowledge and attitudes about the vaccine and campaign, their sources of information, and reasons for children missing vaccination were used by the C4D team to adjust communication activities and messages such as which sources of information and community influencers to focus on for the next round, as well as for the routine immunization program. Visits also continued before each subsequent round to identify and address new areas refusing vaccination. Those with a high level of refusals would receive more attention, including additional household visits by an influencer (depending on the reason) and organization of community meetings with community leaders and influencers, than low-resistant areas.

Toward the end of the outbreak response, and in order to strengthen communication activities for the routine immunization program, UNICEF conducted a qualitative study consisting of focus group discussions and in-depth interviews to obtain a deeper understanding of community attitudes toward vaccination and reasons for children not being vaccinated, since responses such as the child being ill or absent may, in fact, mask actual vaccine refusals. The findings led to new strategies, such as partnering with the national pediatrics association, producing a national TV and radio campaign promoting compliance with routine immunization schedule and updating the national communication strategy for the promotion of routine immunization. The effectiveness of communications activities was evident by reviewing independent monitoring data which reported almost universal awareness of the campaign (97%). Findings also show that a high proportion of respondents (90–95%) were knowledgeable about the vaccine used, its benefits, and the target age group for the polio campaigns.

As for where people learned about the vaccination campaigns, IM data from Deir-ez-Zor prior to Round 1 and from Raqqa post Round 2 showed the key role that mosques played in informing people about the campaigns. This is especially the case in Raqqa, where 45% of respondents mentioned mosques as a source of information. Banners and other printed materials were also major information sources. Interpersonal communications from health workers, community leaders, or mobilizers played more of a role in Deir-ez-Zor (mentioned by 19% and 17% of respondents, respectively) than in Raqqa (8% and 6%).

Key Lessons Learned

1. **Outbreak communication interventions could create a programmatic opportunity to boost immunization coverage**. Hence, they should be continued beyond outbreak response phases to address rooted misperceptions and sustain immunization gains during the outbreak phases.
2. **Addressing vaccine hesitancy requires multiple approaches including engagement with health providers and other influencers.** Communication interventions also need to be phased and probably could go beyond the 6 months set timeframe to interrupt polio virus transmission during an outbreak.
3. **The use of factual approach to communicate the polio outbreak messages could sometimes have limited effect.** However, when complemented with messages framed with other approaches such as fear appeal; emotional; or through the use of testimonials, general refusals, and refusals due to doubt of vaccine efficacy were possibly decreasing.
4. One of the unique aspects of Syria's communications response **was the focus on gauging and addressing vaccine hesitancy before the vaccination campaigns took place.** The Syria experience strengthens the argument that vaccine refusal must be addressed from the start to avoid costly setbacks in polio eradication efforts, instead of doing so after a vaccination campaign as an afterthought. As such, it is important to move beyond risk communication and integrate community engagement, to ensure community ownership and continued involvement in preparedness and response.
5. The experience in Syria also confirms the lessons learned from GPEI concerning **the critical role of community mobilizers and influencers.** Members of the Social Mobilization Network conducted household visits and tracked refusals,

which has built trust at the community level, and played a pivotal role. These experiences in Syria as well as in other countries highlight the importance of engaging community mobilizers who come from the same communities they are working in, have similar ethnic and religious backgrounds, and understand the cultural norms and mindset of the community. Perception, trust, and positive interpersonal communication between communities and healthcare workers are essential to making strides.

6. A critical lesson from a joint WHO/UNICEF review of the 2017 outbreak response in Syria flagged **the important role of the support of local leadership and influencers, particularly medical practitioners,** in ensuring higher uptake of the vaccine (first joint review meeting report). This was also found to be the case in India during its polio eradication campaigns; in two states alone, more than 49,000 community influencers, including health practitioners, teachers, religious leaders, and others, were engaged in actively supporting the campaigns (Deutsch et al., 2017). Like in Syria, community and tribal leaders played an especially active role in supporting polio SIAs and using mosques to announce the campaigns in several countries. Religious leaders in remote and tribal areas of Pakistan, for example, were credited with reducing vaccine refusals for religious reasons by 38% over a 2-month period in 2007 (Waisbord et al., 2010), while the engagement of Muslim leaders in Uttar Pradesh's western region was believed to have made a critical contribution to the reduction to near zero of Muslim children who had not received at least two polio vaccine doses from 2002 to 2004 (Obregón et al., 2009). As a further lesson learned, these community influencers and leaders in Syria also played a key role in monitoring public attitudes toward the polio campaigns throughout the response and in minimizing "campaign fatigue" due to multiple vaccination rounds.
7. Finally, the experience in responding to the Syria outbreak also underscores **the importance of having local capacity on the ground who can play a critical role in planning and coordinating communication and social mobilization activities in conflict zones** that are at high risk of polio and other vaccine-preventable disease outbreaks. Having local communication facilitators on the ground and the high regard in which they held by different sides of the conflict, their negotiating skills, knowledge of the local culture and political situation, and ability to think outside of the box were pivotal to the planning and implementation of the C4D activities during the outbreak response. Given the inability of MOH staff and restrictions of UN personnel to travel to these areas, especially during Round 1, these activities would not have taken place without them. Given their key role, three additional C4D-specific facilitators were hired for Phase 2 of the response and continued to support the communications activities for polio campaigns and the routine immunization program in areas affected by the outbreak. As part of their preparedness plans, countries at high risk of polio outbreaks should have such facilitators already in place in high-risk areas or have a mechanism to recruit and deploy them quickly.

Conclusion

Communication is a critical pillar to the success of any outbreak response. Robust surveillance with early detection, impeccable plans, availability of financial, human, and material resources without effective communication approaches to sensitize communities, religious and community leaders convince the authorities at all levels of the importance of urgent response will lead to sub-optimal coverage resulting in continued transmission and requirement for more resources to response with a possibility of loss of credibility among the communities. Of equal importance is developing **partnerships** from the onset of the outbreak and considering all necessary competencies and replicating these at appropriate lower levels to improve coordination and foster unity of purpose. Lastly, as experienced in both Ukraine and Syria outbreaks, **the use of data** to refine communication approaches, messages, and selection of communication approaches was critical in contributing to the success achieved.

Acknowledgments The authors would like to specially acknowledge the contribution of Ms. Oumou Dao during the drafting process of this chapter. Ms. Dao was Polio Communication for Development intern with UNICEF Regional Office and worked under the guidance of Sahar Hegazi (one of the two authors) while supporting the chapter drafting and while finalizing her master's degree from New York University. Ms. Dao is currently working professionally with the UN Foundation on a related polio program management.

Disclaimer The views expressed in this report are those of the authors and do not necessarily represent the official position of UNICEF or WHO.

References

Curry, D. W., Perry, H. B., Tirmizi, S. N., Goldstein, A. L., & Lynch, M. C. (2014). Assessing the effectiveness of house-to-house visits on routine oral polio immunization completion and tracking of defaulters. *Journal of Health, Population, and Nutrition, 32*(2), 356–366.

Deutsch, N., Singh, P., Singh, V., Curtis, R., & Siddique, A. R. (2017). Legacy of polio-use of India's social mobilization network for strengthening of the universal immunization program in India. *The Journal of Infectious Diseases, 216*(Suppl 1), S260–S266. https://doi.org/10.1093/infdis/jix068

Global Polio Eradication Initiative. (2020). Retrieved from http://polioeradication.org/polio-today/polio-now/this-week/

Independent monitoring surveys for polio outbreak in Ukraine. (n.d.) UNICEF, Ukraine, 2015–2016.

Knowledge, attitude, practice and behavior on immunization & polio. (2014). UNICEF-WHO, Ukraine.

Obregón, R., Chitnis, K., Morry, C., Feek, W., Bates, J., Galway, M., & Ogden, E. (2009). Achieving polio eradication: A review of health communication evidence and lessons learned in India and Pakistan. *Bulletin of the World Health Organization, 87*(8), 624–630. https://doi.org/10.2471/blt.08.060863

Syria cVDPV2 outbreak Situation Report. (n.d.) WHO/UNICEF. Retrieved from http://www.emro.who.int/images/stories/who_unicef_situation_report_14_cvdpv2_outbreak_syria_19.9.2017.pdf?ua=1

Waisbord, S., Shimp, L., Ogden, E. W., & Morry, C. (2010). Communication for polio eradication: Improving the quality of communication programming through real-time monitoring and evaluation. *Journal of Health Communication, 15*(Suppl 1), 9–24. https://doi.org/10.1080/10810731003695375

Weiss, W. M., Choudhary, M., & Solomon, R. (2013). Performance and determinants of routine immunization coverage within the context of intensive polio eradication activities in Uttar Pradesh, India: Social Mobilization Network (SM Net) and Core Group Polio Project (CGPP). *BMC International Health and Human Rights, 13*, 25. https://doi.org/10.1186/1472698X-13-25

Weiss, W. M., Winch, P. J., & Burnham, G. (2009). Factors associated with missed vaccination during mass immunization campaigns. *Journal of Health, Population, and Nutrition, 27*(3), 358–367. https://doi.org/10.3329/jhpn.v27i3.3378

Chapter 5
Complexity and Context of Ebola Virus Disease Preparedness and Response in Eastern and Southern Africa

Charles Kakaire and Ida-Marie Ameda

Contents

Background/Setting the Context

Brief Description of EVD, Its Transmission Pathways, Outbreak Preparedness, and Response

Ebola virus disease (EVD) was first reported in 1976 in concurrent outbreaks in Nzara, present day South Sudan and Yambuku in a village by the River Ebola from which the disease gets its name in the Democratic Republic of the Congo (DRC) (CDC, 2021; WHO, 2021). Since 1976, there have been around 43

C. Kakaire (✉) · I.-M. Ameda
UNICEF East and Southern Africa Regional Office (ESARO), Nairobi, Kenya
e-mail: cnkakaire@unicef.org

E. Manoncourt et al. (eds.), *Communication and Community Engagement in Disease Outbreaks*, https://doi.org/10.1007/978-3-030-92296-2_5

outbreaks in 16 countries (some exported), with the DRC experiencing the majority of outbreaks and over 60% of the reported outbreaks caused by *Zaire ebolavirus,* one of six known Ebola virus species[1] (CDC, 2021; WHO, 2021). EVD re-emergence continues to pose a high public health risk because of the existence of a virus reservoir host *(thought to be the African fruit bat)* particularly in the tropical belt spanning east, central, and west Africa (CDC, 2021; WHO, 2021). Transmission occurs to humans following contact with an infected ill or dead animal. EVD then spreads to other humans by direct contact with (a) infected blood and body fluids of patients and dead bodies, (b) contaminated linen and equipment, (c) within the healthcare setting to/from health workers who do not apply appropriate infection prevention precautions, and (d) new evidence is increasingly pointing to breastmilk and semen of recovered patients as a source of resurgence in communities, while some patients (a few for now) are known to experience reinfection from virus remaining "hidden" in certain parts of the body (MacIntyre & Chughtai, 2016; Nordenstedt et al., 2016; Deen et al., 2017; Bozman et al., 2021).

Most EVD outbreaks have been reported in rural, poor, and neglected communities where people often hunt bushmeat to supplement their nutrition needs, with mobility playing a major role in transmission into urban areas from where outbreaks then spread, including to neighboring/other countries. This was the case in the 2014–2016 west African outbreak as well as in the 2018–2020 outbreak in Northeastern DRC.

Between August 2018 and November 2020, DRC experienced its 10th and 11th EVD outbreaks in North Kivu and Ituri provinces which resulted in cross-border transmission to a border district of Uganda twice (June and August 2019), with the threat of transmission to three other neighboring countries—Burundi, Rwanda, and South Sudan (UNICEF ESARO, 2021). The tenth outbreak was the country's longest outbreak, lasting almost 2 years, and the second largest outbreak in the world following the 2014–2016 EVD outbreak in West Africa. The 11th was a resurgence of the tenth outbreak (Physician's Weekly, 2019). These two outbreaks were also the first to be reported in an active conflict area (UNICEF ESARO, 2021).

Following an assessment by the World Health Organization Regional Office for Africa (WHO AFRO), nine countries neighboring DRC were considered to be at moderate to high risk of spillover of the EVD outbreak and were subsequently considered as "priority countries," as shown in Fig. 5.1. The countries were categorized as priority 1[2] and priority 2[3] based on geographical proximity to the epicenter, volume of cross-border movement and shared transport routes. While all these

[1] The other Ebola virus species include: Bundibugyo, Sudan, with the first two and Zaire responsible for large outbreaks; Taï Forest, Reston, and Bombali (identified in Bats only for now).

[2] Priority 1: Burundi, Rwanda, South Sudan, and Uganda.

[3] Priority 2: Angola, Central African Republic, Congo, the United Republic of Tanzania, and Zambia.

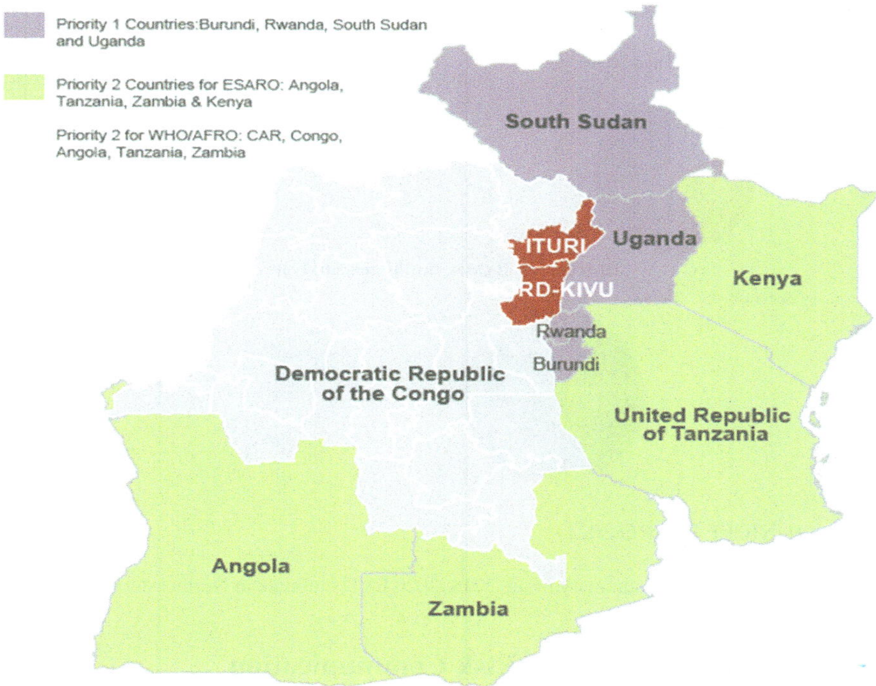

Fig. 5.1 Priority countries for EVD preparedness

countries are member states of WHO/AFRO, they are covered by different UNICEF regional offices (eastern and southern Africa and west and central Africa), this is also the case for a few other regional health partners.

On July 17, 2019, in line with the International Health Regulations (IHR) (2005), the WHO Director-General declared the tenth outbreak a Public Health Emergency of International Concern. This was due to continued intense spread of the disease, including the city of Goma, which serves as a gateway to the rest of East Africa. The fact that the outbreak was occurring in a conflict-affected area also played a role in the declaration, which then prompted intensified scale-up of preparedness actions in both DRC and neighboring Priority 1 countries (IASC, 2019).

The outbreak affected 29 health zones in DRC, mainly in North Kivu, South Kivu, and Ituri Provinces, and by the end of the outbreak, 3470 cases had been reported, with 2287 deaths and 1171 survivors, as illustrated in Fig. 5.2. Approximately 33% of the deaths occurred outside of treatment centers, with 29% occurring among children, 57% among women. Overall, 5% of all cases are believed to have occurred among health workers.

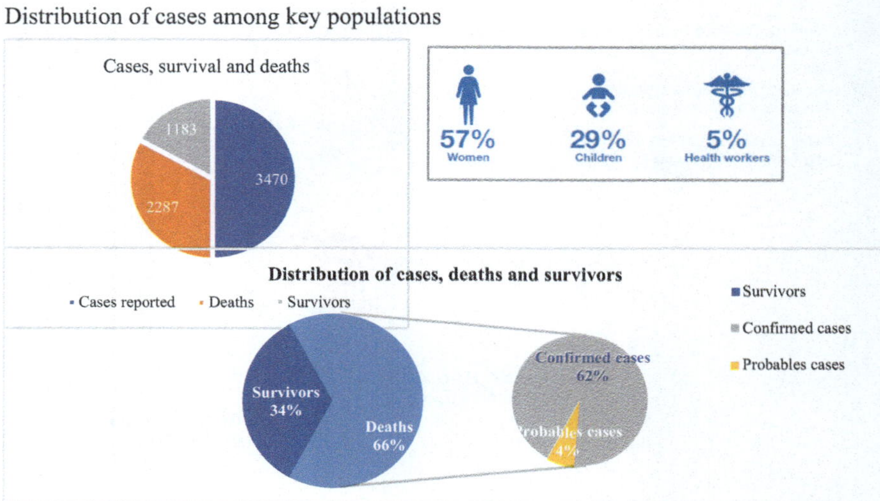

Source: (UNICEF ESARO 2021)

Fig. 5.2 Epidemiological summary of the 2018–2020 EVD outbreak in Northeastern DRC

Scope and Key Actions for Risk Communication and Community Engagement

Risk Communication and Community Engagement (RCCE) is one of the 19 areas assessed in Joint External Evaluations (JEEs), which is the principle tool for assessing country health security core capacities, including countries in conflict (WHO, 2018, 2019). It has been noted that RCCE is an area with suboptimal capacity as evidenced by low JEE scores in half the countries in the WHO African region. The scope within the JEEs is found to be limited to Risk Communication with little to no reflection on Community Engagement processes for outbreak preparedness and response (Talisuna et al., 2019; Garfield et al., 2019). Anecdotal information from countries indicates that the right RCCE stakeholders were not often equally engaged or represented in some IHR processes (such as the JEEs, Intra-Action Reviews, After Action Reviews, and Simulation exercises) as those from other core capacity areas which tended to be skewed toward surveillance and other more "mainstream" health response areas. An After-Action Review (AAR) conducted in Uganda in August 2019 after the end of EVD outbreak declaration enabled an in-depth reflection among RCCE stakeholders of what went well, what did not, and what needed to be improved ahead of the next outbreak. The review assessed the functional capacity of each of the response pillars to detect and respond to an EVD event. From the RCCE pillar, the AAR identified community engagement and availability of communication materials as best practices but identified limited integration of RCCE into the rest of the response (MoH Uganda, 2019).

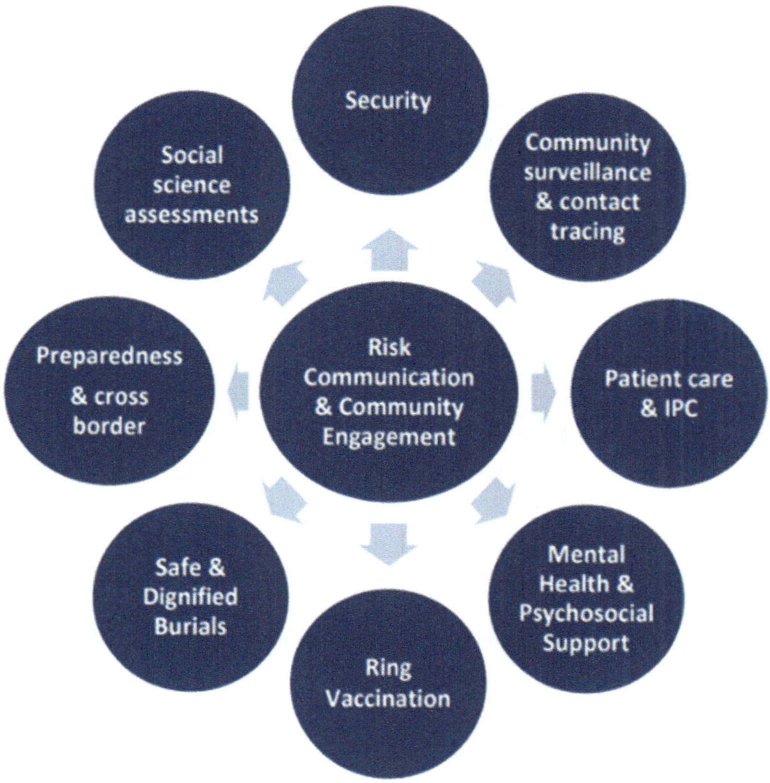

Fig. 5.3 Integration of RCCE principles in all pillars of EVD response (Reprinted with permission from WHO, UNICEF and IFRC. (2018). Risk Communication and Community Engagement Preparedness and Readiness Framework: Ebola Response in the Democratic Republic of Congo in North Kivu. Figure 1. https://apps.who.int/iris/handle/10665/275389, licensed under the terms of the Creative Commons Attribution-NonCommercial-ShareAlike 3.0 IGO license (https://creativecommons.org/licenses/by-nc-sa/3.0/igo))

RCCE as a pillar of EVD outbreak preparedness and response played a key role in contributing to the prevention as well as containment of the outbreak in the countries neighboring the DRC. Under the joint government and WHO-led incident management system, RCCE coordination mechanisms were established in all the priority countries to coordinate the preparedness and response. This ensured that communication strategies and plans were developed, contributing to the broader national preparedness and response plans.

A Risk Communication and Community Engagement framework for EVD developed by WHO, IFRC, and UNICEF provided the guidance for country preparedness and readiness efforts (WHO, UNICEF and IFRC, 2018). The framework in Fig. 5.3 outlines key activities and considerations for intervention areas and also highlighted the linkages between the RCCE response pillar with other technical areas including mental health and psychosocial support, community surveillance and contact tracing, safe and dignified burials, patient care, infection prevention and control, vaccination, and cross-border movement (WHO, 2018).

Under the framework, key interventions were defined for each phase of the preparedness and readiness, including specific actions for priority high-risk groups.

While each of the priority countries adapted preparedness and readiness activities as described in the framework, general intervention categories focused on coordination, evidence generation/formative research, social science research, mass media and communication materials development, social mobilization and community engagement, and collection and analysis of community feedback. Table 5.1 highlights some of the main activities undertaken under each of the above work streams in the respective priority countries.

A Reflection of the Role Played by Context, Culture, Trust, Complexity, and Rights in EVD Preparedness and Response

As noted in previous chapters, culture, rights, complexity, and context play a major role in the response to emergencies. In this chapter, we describe with examples how each of the concepts played a key role in the EVD preparedness and response efforts. For best linkages, we refer to a conceptual model that was used to inform the response.

Context and Complexity

Although the EVD outbreak in West Africa between 2014 and 2016 highlighted the risks of multi-country transmission due to intense cross-border movement, a key lesson learned from the 2018–2020 DRC outbreak was the importance of multi-country cross-border collaboration in outbreak risk mitigation. North Kivu province (DRC), the epicenter of the 2018 outbreak, shares borders with five Eastern Africa countries with frequent cross-border movement related to trade, farming, healthcare, and social activities (Aceng et al., 2020). Understanding how people move within and across borders is critical to understanding how diseases are transmitted and subsequently informing targeted response. It is indeed in this spirit that the International Health Regulations were developed. In DRC, South Sudan, Burundi, and Uganda, the International Organization for Migration (IOM) mapped and analyzed people's mobility trends and dynamics, allowing responders including the risk communication and community engagement pillar to identify hotspots for targeted RCCE intervention, and informing decision-making processes (IOM, 2020). In DRC, a social science cell (CASS) was established to provide a better understanding of the outbreak dynamics to support evidence-based decision-making (UNICEF, 2018). Established as an operational research unit, CASS provided

Table 5.1 Overview of RCCE preparedness and readiness actions for EVD in selected ESA countries

	Country updates				
RCCE work area	Burundi	Rwanda	South Sudan	Tanzania	Uganda
Coordination	National EVD communications subcommission and subcommittees activated at province and district levels, bimonthly meetings of RCCE partners held, and standard operating procedures for EVD RCCE developed	National EVD RCCE working group activated with weekly meetings, and standard operating procedures for EVD RCCE developed	National EVD RCSMCE working group subcommittee activated, weekly meetings held, and standard operating procedures for EVD RCCE developed	RCCE working group activated, biweekly coordination meetings held, and standard operating procedures for EVD RCCE developed	National RCCE working group as well as district and subcounty task forces activated in high-risk districts, weekly coordination meetings held—turned daily during outbreak response, and standard operating procedures for viral hemorrhagic fevers exist
Evidence generation	Knowledge Attitudes and Practice (KAP) surveys conducted in high-risk regions, social science evidence review undertaken to understand cross-border dynamics between Burundi and Democratic Republic of the Congo	KAP surveys in high-risk districts, social science evidence review undertaken to understand cross-border dynamics between Rwanda and Democratic Republic of the Congo	KAP survey conducted in high-risk regions, two social science evidence review undertaken focusing on (1) cross-border dynamics between South Sudan, Uganda, and Democratic Republic of the Congo and (2) bushmeat trade in the border areas of South Sudan and DRC	KAP survey conducted in three high-risk regions with one anthropological study focused on two of the three high-risk regions	Two KAP surveys conducted in high-risk districts, an anthropological study and social science evidence review to understand cross-border dynamics between Uganda and Democratic Republic of the Congo

(continued)

Table 5.1 (continued)

	Country updates				
RCCE work area	Burundi	Rwanda	South Sudan	Tanzania	Uganda
Communication materials	Variety of Information Education and Communication materials including posters, banners, leaflets, job aids, flip charts, and fact sheets for schools produced and distributed in all high-risk locations. A workshop held with representatives from high-risk districts in Uganda to review, revise, and translate materials/messages				
Mass media	Radio messages, talk shows, and call-in programs on EVD	EVD song and video produced with popular artists, radio messages and public service announcement, outdoor LED screen displays in Kigali and border towns, community radio station in border towns, live streaming of roadshows and other mobilization events as well as radio drama series	Radio messages and public service announcements	Radio and television messages, *The Story of Ebola* animation video recorded on flash drives and distributed through public transport, local cinemas, churches, and schools. Journalists' training on EVD reporting	Radio talk shows with direct involvement of technical staff and influential community members, television commercials, radio jingles
Social mobilization and community engagement	Engagement of religious leaders	Community engagement through community health workers, faith-based organizations, and during *Umuganda* (national community workday)	Direct engagement through the Integrated Community Mobilization Network (ICMN) and with various religious groups	Community health worker engagements and through partnership with Tanzania Red Cross Society	Mobilization and engagement through community health workers, and red cross and NGO volunteers
Community feedback	Radio and toll-free line	Toll-free line and community radio with call-back logs	Rumor tracking through the ICMN and toll-free lines	Rumor tracking through the National Health Management Information System	U-Report (mobile phone platform) dashboards, Uganda Red Cross Society volunteers, radio talk shows, community meetings

real-time integrated analysis of community dynamics to influence decision-making of response actors involved in the response. With a core team of researchers, CASS conducted rapid studies to better understand and explain the dynamics around EVD and its impact on the communities and community health (UNICEF, 2018). In their fourth research brief on barriers to healthcare seeking during the DRC Ebola outbreak, CASS identified several factors including fear of being sent to an Ebola treatment center (ETC), mistrust of healthcare workers, fear of contracting Ebola at a healthcare facility, and perceptions of reduced quality of care (CASS, 2020). In the preparedness countries, rapid social science evidence reviews undertaken to understand the unique cross-border dynamics revealed distinct and contextual factors that influenced the behaviors as well as preparedness interventions (Bedford, 2019; Pendle et al., 2019). Issues of language, channels of communication, types, and schedules of economic activities were established to determine community engagement activities; for example, in Uganda this was done through collaboration between the national RCCE pillar and District Health Promotion Officers via face-to-face meetings at the national level as well as field supportive supervision and deployments. While some of these factors identified had little to no linkages to knowledge and awareness about EVD, an analysis and understanding of their contexts with a view to address them was critical, as they were likely to considerably contribute to delays in healthcare seeking by people with suspected Ebola. Dialogues conducted with various groups including youth, women and community leaders in various locations ensured constant dissemination of information about the various aspects of EVD, including the collection and response to community feedback. The deployment of Red Cross volunteers from the national societies across the preparedness countries ensured constant engagement of people on the move at the respective points of entry. With an estimated daily traffic of over 90,000 people crossing the Rwanda/DRC's border, a community radio serving the Rubavu cross-border market provided the needed channel for dissemination of EVD preparedness messages across the border. This was complemented with outdoor LED screens fixed at border points used to broadcast and diversify messaging seen by the thousands of transient people crossing the borders each day (UNICEF, 2019).

Trust and the EVD Preparedness/Response

Trust has many dimensions. While the concept has been defined by (UNICEF and IFRC, 2020) as a firm belief in the reliability and integrity of a person or institution, earlier definitions expanded its meaning to include not only a firm belief in the reliability but also truth, and the ability or strength of someone or something (IFRC and UNICEF, 2020). Regardless of the definition, one thing is clear; trust is the cornerstone of community engagement, be it trust in healthcare providers, community trust in government institutions and healthcare systems, public trust in communication sources and channels), and even more pronounced recently, the trust in COVID-19 vaccines (Alonge et al., 2019). While trust and trust building is a widely recognized concept pertinent to engagement, it remains elusive, and one reason for this is its complexity (Wilkins, 2018). The role of mistrust has been identified as a driver of low community engagement with the Ebola response (Ozawa & Stack, 2013; Carrión Martín et al., 2016; Ryan et al., 2019). Evidence from several CASS studies showed that communities in DRC had a high mistrust for Health Care Workers (HCWs) and foreign responders especially related to perceived high remunerations (CASS, 2019). There was a general belief that from the start of the outbreak, everyone who visited a health center for any health condition would be diagnosed with Ebola and subsequently sent to an Ebola Treatment Center leading to a financial reward for HCWs. This lack of trust fueled by the HCW's inability to speak the local languages was a major barrier to health-seeking behaviors. There was a broader mistrust in the authorities by the affected communities, long disenfranchised, and with the poorest of health and nutrition indicators, with very little concerted effort to address them. Armed with information on the context in the DRC preparedness countries instituted mechanisms to ensure that community trust was built. Social mobilizers who undertook outreaches were recruited from the high-risk districts, and RCCE preparedness activities were coordinated through subnational RCCE mechanisms. The engagement of local leaders as well as religious and traditional leaders in RCCE activities, including participation in radio talk shows in the high-risk locations ensured that community engagement and outreaches were undertaken by individuals familiar to and who were familiar with their own communities (UNICEF, 2020). Beyond RCCE, there were efforts to address other health, nutrition, and social service gaps through "Ebola Plus," an expansion of the response to address health, nutrition, and water and sanitation gaps in the affected communities. As with all other interventions, trust was an essential element for gaining community acceptance of both the messages and the preparedness interventions. Indeed, as noted in a DRC study by Vinck and colleagues, there was a correlation between trust in government authorities and compliance with government EVD control measures during the 2019 EVD outbreak response in North Kivu, DRC (Vinck et al., 2019).

Culture and the EVD Preparedness/Response

Cultural norms around livelihoods, religious beliefs, burial practice, caretaking practices, and health beliefs have been known to influence uptake of public health measures and are particularly important during public health emergencies where they can easily propagate disease. We look at some specific practices which had implications on preparedness efforts.

Burial Practices

Across different part of Africa and in the four countries, burial rituals are a vital aspect of local culture across different regions and religions (Schmidt-Sane et al., 2021). It is noted that there are prescribed and locally meaningful practices that are believed to bear influence on an individual, with some beliefs that the souls of the dead cannot rest well and will always live to haunt the family unless these rituals are performed correctly (Bedford, 2018). Certain burial rituals and practices are also notably different between religions. An important aspect of preparedness was understanding these practices especially as in many societies, the traditional practices around burial include close contact with the deceased. Ripoll and others note that the acceptability of these approaches to family members as an alternative means of honoring the dead is uncertain, but evidence from previous outbreaks has shown people to be generally pragmatic, adaptable, and willing to change practices if the need is understood and acceptable alternatives are agreed (Ripoll et al., 2019). Given the close physical contact with the bodies during traditional and religious burial practices, increasing community members' knowledge of the importance of safe burials of suspected EVD cases and supervised burials for probable cases was a central part of preparedness efforts in the priority countries. In Uganda, burial practices differ by culture and religion, however, certain practices appear to be similar such as body preparation, holding of vigils and burial on ancestral lands (Mafigiri & Schmidt-Sane, 2019). To ensure that their relatives were buried in accordance with cultural practice, sometimes families transported them on a boda boda (motorcycle taxi), disguised as a passenger on a wicker chair; beyond EVD, the rider/transporters noted that it was an option that families sometimes used when they could not afford to hire a vehicle to transport the body (Mafigiri & Schmidt-Sane, 2019).

Treatment Seeking

Treatment decisions across different communities vary and are often influenced by perceptions about the cause of illness, severity, or complexity of beliefs (SSHAP, 2019a). Financial and non-financial barriers are known to influence decisions regarding when, where, and from whom to seek healthcare. Issues such as distance from home to the health facilities, availability of transport and the level of trust in health providers and treatment options contribute and influence the care seeking. A biomedical diagnosis is not a substitute for alternative treatment, as other options are sought either consecutively or in parallel, more so for chronic diseases and repeated episodes of sickness. As a result, people with EVD can potentially transmit disease to drug store/stall attendants, herbalists, and health workers because they consult all three—this was noted in North Kivu where private health practitioners, herbalists, and drug store attendants were engaged in RCCE, requested to refer patients to the treatment center and also prioritized for EVD vaccination to lower risk of contracting and transmitting disease themselves. In Uganda, an anthropological study found that some communities contacted drug stores or traditional healers first because they were cheaper and appeared to offer immediate relief (Mafigiri & Schmidt-Sane, 2019). They noted that efforts to engage with traditional healers met with varying levels of success, from meeting "no shows" to full on engagement including with healers insisting on temperature screening and hand hygiene before consultations.

One of the key features of the EVD preparedness efforts was related to perceptions about treatment centers especially around the construction of Ebola isolation and treatment units. While these are the norm in typical outbreak settings, WHO noted that establishment of these in communities where there were no active cases was met with mixed feelings (WHO AFRO, 2021). The rapid construction of temporary facilities which were specific to a disease not experienced before contributed to the community suspicion. In response, open days initiated to allow community members to visit the Ebola Treatment Units prior to their use were helpful in demystifying the suspicions, allaying fears, curiosity, and doubt within the community.

Gendered Roles and EVD Infection

Previous studies have attributed higher EVD infection rates among women (and teenage girls) to culturally prescribed caregiving roles (Mühlberger et al., 2015; WHO AFRO, 2021). Often women provide care within the household, and it is generally expected that they attend to all patients within the household, and if they are admitted to a facility, their family offers support and care during this period. These lessons learned demonstrated that understanding social norms and caregiving practices is critical in an effective EVD response (Harman, 2016). Obtaining a comprehensive understanding of caregiving practices, gender roles, and responsibilities during an EVD outbreak requires an understanding of the social and cultural context of the outbreak and proposing a risk mitigation approach for example referrals to the treatment center with scheduled and safe family support and/or visits.

Human Rights in EVD Preparedness

As noted in the first chapter, the increase in disease outbreaks and public health emergencies of international concern, and the accompanying restrictions that come with them brings human rights issues at the center of preparedness and response efforts. Meier and colleagues writing about public health and human rights noted that instances where the two fields have shared focus, the tendency is to utilize rights-based approaches which emphasize principles of "individual empowerment, community participation, and government accountability" (Meier et al., 2018).

Often public health emergencies recur in places where communities are neglected—both hard to reach and underserved, referred to elsewhere in public health programs as areas "at the end of the road." Using a rights-based and community informed lens in the response is not just recommended, it is the only way to make real progress. During the DRC outbreak, a rapid community feedback mechanism was established by IFRC to collect near real-time community insights to inform the response (IFRC C, 2020). Through their local network of community volunteers, community concerns, rumors and questions were captured, compiled, and analyzed on an ongoing basis to inform response actions. In several social science briefs, for example, it was clear that residents of Goma faced many livelihood challenges, and despite the existence of an EVD outbreak, Ebola was not their main concern, but rather other issues such as food security, neighborhood crime and insecurity, and health challenges such as malaria, typhoid, and cholera (SSHAP, 2019b). This led to the initiation of Ebola plus where communication messages were framed to ensure alignment with other challenges, such as increased handwashing being helpful in reducing the risk of typhoid, cholera, and related enteric illnesses as well as Ebola. In Uganda, communities in Rwenshama fishing village on Lake Edward, which borders DRC, reported punitive measures including breaking boats for illegal fishing, which then compromised their ability to repay business loans, with some women indicating that "they wished they could die of Ebola" instead (Mafigiri & Schmidt-Sane, 2019). While indirectly linked to the response, this loss of livelihood which the community found to be unjust treatment of them by government, contributed to a negative perception of the response.

Implications for Future Preparedness/Response

The prolonged period of community awareness for Ebola prevention resulted in a state of message fatigue which So and colleagues described as state of being exhausted and tired of prolonged exposure to similarly themed messages (So et al., 2017). This called for innovative strategies around messages, format, and delivery platforms to ensure that audiences were kept engaged while maintaining a high perception of risk during preparedness. So and colleagues note that this fatigue contributes to two types of reactions notably, reactance and disengagement, which are likely to reduce the audience intention to adopt the recommended behaviors advocated for in the message. RCCE interventions for prolonged health emergencies such as the current COVID-19 outbreak will require concerted efforts to maintain audience engagement as fatigue is a likely barrier to effective health communication.

Social science research should be incorporated into RCCE preparedness efforts to help understand the unique contextual and social dynamics (beyond knowledge), in order to inform strategy and message design. Operational briefs produced during the DRC EVD outbreak were used to inform the response on the different local social and cultural contexts of outbreak-affected areas which in turn helped shape the response measures (SSHAP, 2019a). Similarly, an anthropological study conducted in the high-risk districts of Uganda revealed critical community issues, which influenced the adoption of, and adherence to preparedness efforts.

Planning and implementation of outbreak preparedness interventions should follow a scenario-based approach, clearly outlining key activities to be undertaken during each phase of preparedness. Such activities should be complemented with clear guidance for a nuanced transition of activities between preparedness and response (UNICEF ESARO, 2021).

The 2014/2015 EVD outbreaks in West Africa, the recent DRC outbreak and the current COVID-19 pandemic have all revealed an increased need for strengthened cross-border collaboration and coordination for RCCE and other pillars between neighboring countries. The free movement of people and the unique geographical and sociocultural dynamics of border communities calls for specific contextualized strategies, to address their unique contexts.

Conclusion

RCCE preparedness, although challenging due to lack of political and funding commitments as well as potential fatigue among the communities/people, should be prioritized as a core element of outbreak preparedness and response. Despite the challenges, some generic activities should be prioritized as part of standard preparedness efforts. These could include, but not limited to the collection and analysis of social data to understand the local contextual dynamics, compilation of roster of personnel with the requisite skills, a media landscape analysis to understand the common channels of communication including language preferences, mapping of RCCE partners by location and area of specialization, and establishment and composition of RCCE coordination mechanisms at both national and subnational levels. These standard activities should be complemented with the establishment and training a network of local social mobilizers by location to support early detection and early action to outbreaks as first responders. In his paper on the role of communication in building resilience, Skuse (2015) noted that information and communication can be considered core "protective assets" in any struggle against stress, shocks, and fragility. Engaging communities early and providing them with the basic information and skills about the spread of diseases, how to take preventative actions and ensuring that the necessary communication mechanisms to ensure timely information sharing are in place, are all critical elements of preparedness. Putting these in place will have significant impact on the mitigation and management of the next outbreak of "disease X," including the subsequent waves of the current COVID-19 pandemic.

Disclaimer While the Ebola virus disease (EVD) preparedness and response were based on UNICEF guidance, the views expressed in this chapter are of the writers and do not reflect UNICEF's official position.

References

Aceng, J. R., Ario, A. R., Muruta, A. N., et al. (2020). Uganda's experience in Ebola virus disease outbreak preparedness, 2018–2019. *Global Health, 16*, 24. https://doi.org/10.1186/s12992-020-00548-5

Alonge, O., Sonkarlay, S., Gwaikolo, W., et al. (2019). Understanding the role of community resilience in addressing the Ebola virus disease epidemic in Liberia: A qualitative study (community resilience in Liberia). *Global Health Action, 12*, 1662682. https://doi.org/10.1080/16549716.2019.1662682

Bedford, J. (2019, April 2019). Rwanda—DRC cross border dynamics.

Bedford, J. (2018). Key considerations: Burial, funeral and mourning practices in Équateur Province, DRC.

Bozman, C. M., Fallah, M., Sneller, M. C., et al. (2021). Increased likelihood of detecting Ebola virus RNA in semen by using sample pelleting. *Emerging Infectious Diseases Journal, 27*(4), 1239–1241. https://doi.org/10.3201/eid2704.204175

Carrión Martín, A. I., Derrough, T., Honomou, P., et al. (2016). Social and cultural factors behind community resistance during an Ebola outbreak in a village of the Guinean Forest region, February 2015: A field experience. *International Health, 8*, 227–229. https://doi.org/10.1093/inthealth/ihw018

CDC. (2021). *Ebola virus disease*. Retrieved May 2, 2021, from https://www.cdc.gov/vhf/ebola/index.html

Cellule d'Analyse en Sciences Sociales (CASS). (2020). https://www.socialscienceinaction.org/resources/socialscience-support-covid-19-barriers-healthcare-seeking/. Accessed 31 December 2021.

Deen, G. F., Broutet, N., Xu, W., et al. (2017). Ebola RNA persistence in semen of Ebola virus disease survivors—Final report. *New England Journal of Medicine, 377*, 1428–1437. https://doi.org/10.1056/NEJMoa1511410

Garfield, R., Bartee, M., & Mayigane, L. N. (2019). Validating joint external evaluation reports with the quality of outbreak response in Ethiopia, Nigeria and Madagascar. *BMJ Global Health, 4*, e001655. https://doi.org/10.1136/bmjgh-2019-001655

Harman, S. (2016). Ebola, gender and conspicuously invisible women in global health governance. *Third World Quarterly, 37*, 524–541. https://doi.org/10.1080/01436597.2015.1108827

IASC. (2019). *Key messages on the IASC system-wide scale-up activation for the Ebola response*. Retrieved from https://interagencystandingcommittee.org/iasc-transformative-agenda/news-public/key-messages-iasc-system-wide-scale-activation-ebola-response

IFRC and UNICEF. (2020). Building trust within and across communities for health emergency preparedness, July 2020—World. *ReliefWeb*. Retrieved May 21, 2021, from https://reliefweb.int/report/world/building-trust-within-and-across-communities-health-emergency-preparedness-july-2020

IFRC C. (2020). Real-time Ebola community feedback mechanism, 4.

IOM. (2020). 5 ways IOM helped defeat Ebola in the eastern regions' urban spaces and borders—Democratic Republic of the Congo. *ReliefWeb*. Retrieved May 12, 2021, from https://reliefweb.int/report/democratic-republic-congo/democratic-republic-congo-5-ways-iom-helped-defeat-ebola-eastern

MacIntyre, C. R., & Chughtai, A. A. (2016). Recurrence and reinfection—A new paradigm for the management of Ebola virus disease. *International Journal of Infectious Diseases, 43*, 58–61. https://doi.org/10.1016/j.ijid.2015.12.011

Mafigiri, D., & Schmidt-Sane, M. M. (2019) *Strengthening community linkages to Ebola virus disease (EVD) outbreak preparedness in Uganda*. Retrieved from https://www.unicef.org/uganda/reports/strengthening-community-linkages-ebola-virus-disease-evd-outbreak-preparedness-uganda

Meier, B. M., Evans, D. P., Kavanagh, M. M., et al. (2018). Human rights in public health. *Health and Human Rights, 20*, 85–91.
MoH Uganda. (2019, June). Uganda after action review EVD June outbreak (unpublished).
Mühlberger, E., Roy, D., Scully, P., et al. (2015). Ebola and its discontents. *Catalyst: Feminism, Theory, Technoscience, 1*, 1–14. https://doi.org/10.28968/cftt.v1i1.28822
Nordenstedt, H., Bah, E. I., de la Vega, M.-A., et al. (2016). Ebola virus in breast Milk in an Ebola virus–positive mother with twin babies, Guinea, 2015. *Emerging Infectious Diseases, 22*, 759–760. https://doi.org/10.3201/eid2204.151880
Ozawa, S., & Stack, M. L. (2013). Public trust and vaccine acceptance-international perspectives. *Human Vaccines & Immunotherapeutics, 9*, 1774–1778. https://doi.org/10.4161/hv.24961
Pendle, N., Marko, F. D., & Gercama, I., & Bedford, J. (2019). Key considerations: Cross-border dynamics between south Sudan and DRC.
Physician's Weekly. (2019). First Ebola relapse recorded in Congo outbreak, WHO says. *Physician's Weekly*. Retrieved March 30, 2021, from https://www.physiciansweekly.com/first-ebola-relapse-recorded/
Ripoll, et al. (2019). Social science in epidemics: Ebola virus disease lessons learned—Democratic Republic of the Congo. *ReliefWeb*. Retrieved May 12, 2021, from https://reliefweb.int/report/democratic-republic-congo/social-science-epidemics-ebola-virus-disease-lessons-learned
Ryan, M. J., Giles-Vernick, T., & Graham, J. E. (2019). Technologies of trust in epidemic response: Openness, reflexivity and accountability during the 2014-2016 Ebola outbreak in West Africa. *BMJ Global Health, 4*, e001272. https://doi.org/10.1136/bmjgh-2018-001272
Schmidt-Sane, M., Nielsen, J., Chikombero, M., et al. (2021). Gendered care at the margins: Ebola, gender, and caregiving practices in Uganda's border districts. *Global Public Health* 1–13. https://doi.org/10.1080/17441692.2021.1879895
Skuse, A. (2015). Resilience and the role of information and communication, unpublished paper.
So, J., Kim, S., & Cohen, H. (2017). Message fatigue: Conceptual definition, operationalization, and correlates. *Communication Monographs, 84*, 5–29. https://doi.org/10.1080/03637751.2016.1250429
SSHAP. (2019a). *Updates on DR Congo Ebola outbreak 2019-2020—Social science in humanitarian action platform*. Retrieved May 21, 2021, from https://www.socialscienceinaction.org/updates-dr-congo-ebola-outbreak-2019/
SSHAP. (2019b). *Ebola preparedness and readiness in Goma, DRC—Social science in humanitarian action platform*. Retrieved June 24, 2021, from https://opendocs.ids.ac.uk/opendocs/bitstream/handle/20.500.12413/14422/SSHAP_Ebola_Key_Considerations_Goma.pdf?sequence=1&isAllowed=y
Talisuna, A., Yahaya, A. A., Rajatonirina, S. C., et al. (2019). Joint external evaluation of the International Health Regulation (2005) capacities: Current status and lessons learnt in the WHO African region. *BMJ Global Health, 4*, e001312. https://doi.org/10.1136/bmjgh-2018-001312
UNICEF. (2018). *Social sciences analytics cell (CASS)*. Retrieved May 21, 2021, from https://www.unicef.org/drcongo/en/social-sciences-analytics-cell
UNICEF. (2019, October). UNICEF Rwanda humanitarian situation report no. 3 (Ebola).
UNICEF ESARO. (2020). Risk communication and community engagement for Ebola virus disease preparedness and response lessons learnt and recommendations from Burundi, Rwanda, South Sudan, Tanzania and Uganda 27-28 January 2020.
UNICEF ESARO. (2021). *UNICEF Eastern and Southern Africa Regional Office (2020) Ebola virus disease preparedness and response in priority eastern and southern Africa countries 2018–2020, Nairobi*. UNICEF.
Vinck, P., Pham, P. N., Bindu, K. K., et al. (2019). Institutional trust and misinformation in the response to the 2018–19 Ebola outbreak in North Kivu, DR Congo: A population-based survey. *Lancet Infectious Diseases, 19*, 529–536. https://doi.org/10.1016/S1473-3099(19)30063-5
WHO. (2021). *Ebola virus disease factsheet*. Retrieved May 2, 2021, from https://www.who.int/news-room/fact-sheets/detail/ebola-virus-disease

WHO. (2018). *Joint external evaluation tool: International health regulations (2005), second edition*. World Health Organization.
WHO. (2019). *Guidance document for joint external evaluation in special context countries*. World Health Organization.
WHO AFRO. (2021). *EVD technical coordination platform—Emergency preparedness and response*. Technical report 2019 to 2020 (unpublished).
WHO, UNICEF and IFRC. (2018). Risk communication and community engagement preparedness and readiness framework: Ebola response in the Democratic Republic of Congo in North Kivu.
Wilkins, C. H. (2018). Effective engagement requires trust and being trustworthy. *Med Care, 56*, S6–S8. https://doi.org/10.1097/MLR.0000000000000953

Chapter 6
Ebola in Sierra Leone: Leveraging Community Assets to Strengthen Preparedness and Response

Lawrence Sao Babawo, Foday Mahmoud Kamara, Esther Yei Mokuwa, Gelejimah Alfred Mokuwa, Marion Baby-May Nyakoi, and Paul Richards

Contents

Setting the Context

Brief Description of the Outbreak and Response

A deadly mystery illness with symptoms of severe fever and vomiting began to circulate in two villages in Kissi Teng chiefdom, Kailahun District, eastern Sierra Leone in March 2014 (Richards, 2016). These villages are adjacent to a busy ferry point for foot passengers on the River Moa linking Guinea to Sierra Leone. A nurse who had been treating private patients in Guinea was brought to the health center in Foindu (Kissi Teng chiefdom) and referred to the Government Hospital in Kenema on or about May 21. She made it only as far as the health center at Daru (Jawei

L. S. Babawo · F. M. Kamara · M. B.-M. Nyakoi · P. Richards (✉)
Njala University, Freetown, Sierra Leone
e-mail: paul@akaresearch.co.uk

E. Y. Mokuwa
Wageningen University & Research, Wageningen, The Netherlands

G. A. Mokuwa
Eastern Technical University, Kenema, Sierra Leone

E. Manoncourt et al. (eds.), *Communication and Community Engagement in Disease Outbreaks*, https://doi.org/10.1007/978-3-030-92296-2_6

chiefdom) where she died. Blood tests subsequently confirmed Ebola. A herbalist in Kissy Teng also tested positive for Ebola, and the Ministry of Health and Sanitation reported the presence of the disease in the country to the WHO on May 25, 2014.

Widely attended funerals of the herbalist and nurse—both prominent persons in their communities—triggered further infections. Cases reached Kenema Government Hospital, the largest facility of its kind in the eastern part of the country. The hospital was not equipped to handle the disease, resulting in a large nosocomial outbreak among patients. Sick people shunned the hospital and sought treatment from herbal practitioners (Richards et al., 2015). This distributed the disease to inaccessible locations in the countryside where further prevention proved challenging. Cases then soon reached the capital Freetown, spreading rapidly along a main road system much improved by investment following a decade long civil war of the 1990s.

By August 2014, the infection was increasing countrywide at an alarming rate, matched by equally rapid increases in Guinea and Liberia, and an international alarm was raised. The WHO declared the West African Ebola outbreak a Public Health Emergency of International Concern (PHEIC) on August 8, 2014, triggering a major international response.

Yet, even as new infections emerged in other parts of the country, the outbreaks in Kissi Teng and Jawei chiefdoms in Kailahun District (accounting for over 400 laboratory-confirmed cases) were showing signs of responding to control. Many international Ebola responders were too new to the country to grasp fully what that might signify.

Scope and Key Actions: An Over-centralized Initial Response

The established Freetown-based international agencies were slow to assess the news of outbreak in Kailahun in late May, in part due to difficulties at the country office of WHO. A group of international advisors, led by a senior UN diplomat, the country director of the Food and Agriculture Organization (FAO), finally reached Kailahun at the end of June 2014, 5 weeks after the outbreak was first declared, and reported a strong local response, involving community mobilization, backed by traditional rulers, police, army, and local officials of various ministries.

The benefits of this local response were soon apparent. In July and August, cases in Kailahun slowed to a trickle, with a near complete ending of transmission in September–October, even as the epidemic was peaking in other parts of the country.

New language was invented to cover the situation in the daily dashboard of the National Ebola Response Commission, areas where Ebola transmission had ceased were henceforth known as "silent districts." But little thought was given to the message from the "silent districts". By October, a large international response was gearing up in Freetown, preoccupied with its own coordination (Walsh & Johnson, 2018). The message that people on the ground might contribute an important understanding of their own to the response was overlooked.

The international agencies emphasized top-down command-and-control. This was apparent not only in the involvement of the national army and medical personnel from the British army but also in the rapid establishment of large-scale Ebola treatment centers (ETC), typically capable of handling several hundred patients, in which all movement in and out was subject to the strictest of controls to manage infection risks. Staff breaking the rules were subject to prompt dismissal. This included foreign volunteers.

ETC proved highly controversial. Initially, they offered only palliative care and were widely seen by Sierra Leoneans and by some their staff as hospices—places where patients went to die with dignity rather than hope of recovery. Initial case fatality rates (CFR) were as high as 70%, and thus at the outset there were few survivors to offer a positive story (Richards et al., 2019). Matters improved when dehydration therapy was safely introduced from October 2014 (Lamontagne et al., 2014). This reduced ETC death rates by half or more and increased the flow of survivors back to communities.[1]

There was still a problem, however. Several of these large ETC had been built behind instead of ahead of the advance of the epidemic. This meant that local need tended to decline even as an ETC was opened, and patients were brought in from further distances (Mokuwa & Maat, 2020). For example, the Red Cross ETC at Nganyahun, 15 km north of Kenema, opened in September 2014, was taking, by December, a large number of patients from Kono and Freetown (150- and 300-km distances).

Distance prevented the flow of information between ETC and communities they served (Richards et al., 2020); not all families know where members who perished in a distant ETC are buried.

There was some improvement in local acceptance of Ebola care when the policy of building triage centers (Community Care Centers, CCC), supported by UKAid and UNICEF, was introduced from November 2014 (Mokuwa & Maat, 2020).

In all, about 55 were built. These were located where case numbers were rising. Families could often walk with a patient to a CCC while symptoms were relatively mild. The patient was tested and, if Ebola positive (E+), transferred to an ETC. Some cases were handled within the CCC itself, which was basically laid out like an ETC, with red and green zones for infection control of E+ patients. Those with other disease were treated and discharged. Small in size, with locally recruited and trained staff, and transparent to families, who were often able to talk through the boundary fence to patients in open-sided tents, CCC were much better accepted by communities than the large and forbidding ETC (Mokuwa & Maat, 2020). The rate of discovery and speed of isolation of Ebola cases improved as a result.

It could be said that the CCCs helped re-localize the response, after initial over-centralization by the international Ebola responders. The same could also be said concerning mobile laboratories, provided by several donors, since these could be

[1] Eventual CFR was as low as 23%, a figure achieved at Kerry Town ETC late on in the epidemic (Haaskjold et al., 2016).

moved around to speed up diagnosis in districts with rising numbers of cases. But both were institutional patches. It is worth asking whether more could have been done to strengthen local responses by explicitly recognizing the key work done by local agents and gearing international support to support these activities. To answer this question requires some consideration of what actually was mobilized in local responses to Ebola in Sierra Leone, which in turn hinges on questions of culture, rights, information, and trust (see Chap. 1, Fig. 1.1), including contributions made by local institutions such as chieftaincy and secret power associations to Ebola governance.

Issues of Culture, Rights, Complexity, and Context

Strengths/Opportunities for Local Level Ebola Response

The Family

Ebola is a disease of social intimacy; it affects those who care for the sick and bury the dead, and in Sierra Leone, this is primarily the responsibility of the family (Richards, 2016).

The family in Sierra Leone is a complex, extended structure. Domestic groups are mainly organized in terms of consanguineous patrilineal connection, tied to cultivation rights over land in a village of origin. Where descent is not the criterion for family linkage, other modes of association come into play. Migrants become attached to families through the institution of strangerhood (recognition of incomers as tenants of household heads with local land rights). The landlord (or "stranger father") then represents the tenant in the public sphere—in legal disputes, for example. Children of parents who have migrated to town are often fostered to village-based family members or contacts, and fostering often forges a lasting social connection, similar to adoption.

In the Ebola epidemic, these extended family linkages came to be associated with long-distance infection risks sometimes puzzling to case finders and external observers. Unexpected outlier cases—new infections in long "silent" districts, for example—were explained by family visits to exchange subsistence goods, to attend important family occasions, or to visit the sick and take part in ceremonies, not least funerals. Something not apparent at first also became increasingly evident—that the Ebola virus survives for extended periods in body fluids—and that Ebola was to an extent a sexually transmitted disease, with network patterns of spread not dissimilar to HIV/AIDS.

If a key requirement of Ebola responses was to understand these, often complex patterns of family attachment, and to anticipate the potential infection risks they posed, from where was this information to be derived?

International responders were not well-informed about patterns of social interaction based on kinship or marriage and had to seek advice from social anthropologists via the Ebola Response Anthropology Platform (ERAP). ERAP also mobilized important information from local experts concerning family networks and infection risks associated with ceremonial, such as funerals, and made these rapidly available through a website (www.ebola-anthropology.net). An achievement of ERAP was to bring family perspectives rapidly within the purview of Ebola responders.[2]

This was only part of the task, however, since a clash of perspectives then became readily apparent. Families emphasized their responsibilities for care and burial. Responders emphasized infection control, sometimes pushing for draconian measures without adequately assessing what this would mean in family terms, and without being able always to provide relevant evidence on risks involved.

One example of this was what to do about the bedding of Ebola cases. Routinely, this was destroyed by burning. This represented a severe loss to a poor family, and compensation was introduced. But the burning angered families, since they thought it unnecessary. Locally, it was argued that "sunning" the bedding before thorough washing would suffice. Where they could, people did this on the quiet, and no firm evidence of harm ever came to light. Data on how long fomites remained active on bedding after exposure to strong tropical sunlight were (and still are) in short supply.

Burial and Homecare

The biggest source of conflict was undoubtedly the washing of the body at death. This is required for Muslims. Most rural Sierra Leoneans are Muslims, and non-Muslim groups have often adopted Muslim standards on this issue. A certain cultural deafness to Muslim sensitivities was an unfortunate aspect of the international Ebola response in Upper West Africa.

Washing the body of someone who might have died of Ebola was banned. The prohibition admitted no exceptions. Even though few cases in the period 2014–2015 were Ebola deaths, as a proportion of all deaths, there is little doubt that a ban on body washing was proportionate to the high risk involved. But the ban was clumsy because it went too far. It failed to differentiate between corpse handling and funerals. More could have been done to make funerals safer. Faster swab testing, for example, might have released bodies that were not Ebola deaths; and there was probably no need to ban witnesses attending a burial provided they kept clear of the corpse. Banning too much fostered clandestine burial.

Events on the ground—natural experiments, they might be termed—sometimes made clear where opportunities to bring families more fully into the "safe burial" process had been missed. In the early part of the epidemic in Kailahun bodies were buried by volunteers working under the supervision of Paramount Chiefs. There

---

[2] The success of ERAP has been generalized to cover epidemic and pandemic disease threats, along with health and other emergencies, in a similar platform and network model known as the Social Science in Humanitarian Action Platform (SSHAP, www.socialscienceinaction.org).

was no alternative, since the international response was yet to be rolled out. Safety measures were applied in an ad hoc manner as and where protective materials were available. Local observers pointed out that the volunteers improvised their own protection and lived to tell the tale.

Under later rules for safe burial response was often slow, and communities at times decided they had no option but to do the job themselves. Effective performance by community group of volunteers in such cases sometimes led to them being "adopted" by District Ebola Response Committees for training and authorization as official burial teams. The fact that earlier, unauthorized work did not lead to loss of infection control suggests that more could have been done to involve communities in the safe burial process from the outset.

Families also deeply resented what they saw as the heartless dumping of bodies in graves by official burial teams, aided by poles and sticks. They argued that only those who knew and valued the life of the deceased could properly care for the body after death. Being excluded from the actual burial process heightened feelings of distress and social dislocation.

International responders did eventually introduce badly needed reforms. Burial teams were better trained in the need to show respect for the dead. The funeral rules were changed by mandating the participation of an imam or pastor. Family members were invited to witness the event at a distance (WHO, 2014).

There were also changes in official thinking about family care for the sick. Advisors initially feared this would encourage families to keep Ebola cases at home rather than seek care in an ETC. But of necessity homecare happened in more isolated districts, beyond the reach of ambulances and emergency telephones. Moving such patients in these cases (by hammock) probably posed more risks of infection than caring for them in situ.

Requests to publish basic guidance on safe palliative care in such conditions (where, for example, there was no road for an ambulance) were summarily rejected. Later there was a re-think, and in October 2014, the US Centers for Disease Control and Prevention (CDC) issued a poster for Sierra Leone entitled "Taking care of someone with suspected Ebola: what to do while waiting for help" (Richards, 2016, pp. 116–117). This was in effect a homecare protocol. It could have been provided much earlier and might have fostered better cooperation with communities.

Local Leadership

An important aspect of Sierra Leone's Ebola response was the part played by local leadership. The bottom layer of the system of local government comprised the 149 chieftaincies into which provincial Sierra Leone was divided in 2014–2015. The part played by chiefs in Ebola response was crucial. This is because they are a group of officials living day by day with the ordinary people, a consideration of huge importance in addressing what was a family disease.

The origins of local rule by Paramount Chiefs dates from the British colonial occupation. Pre-colonial Sierra Leone was a world shaped by warlord competition. Alliances of local rulers resisted British occupation in the rebellion of 1898. The British then imposed a military occupation, reinforced by building a railway, and sought local persons of influence to rule on their behalf once the rebels had been removed. Paramount Chiefs under the British system of colonial Indirect Rule were elected by representatives of the local land-owning clans, subject to approval by British administrators.[3]

"Paramount," in British colonial usage in Sierra Leone, meant specifically that each chief was paramount in his or her own chiefdom, i.e., no chief could interfere in the affairs of another chiefdom without incurring the wrath of the British overlords. In southern and eastern Sierra Leone, women could be, and were, elected as Paramount Chiefs. Sub-chiefs were then appointed under each Paramount Chief to administer each settlement within a chiefdom. Later, each Paramount chief was advised by a chiefdom council.

The system, while subject to political interference, proved a durable way of maintaining local order, and survived into the period of colonial independence, but fell apart during the decade long civil war in the 1990s. Older chiefs died, sometimes in the fighting and were not replaced; younger chiefs sometimes fled to the security of the towns and lost legitimacy as defenders of their communities. The institution was revived after the civil war of 1991–2002, when chiefs were re-housed and given additional training by a British-funded chiefdom reform project.

Paramount Chiefs are tasked and trained more explicitly to take responsibility for local security and are today required to keep a close eye on a range of potential threats, including disease outbreaks. One Paramount Chief active in the fight against Ebola (Kallon, of Jawei chiefdom, Kailahun District) told us that he reports any disaster to the Office of National Security and any health concerns to the District Health Management Team (DHMT) of the Ministry of Health and Sanitation (interview, Marion Nyakoi, May 20, 2021). Another Paramount Chief proactive in Ebola response (Sovula, of Kamajei chiefdom, Moyamba District) explained that reporting of health issues and disaster management are duties of Paramount Chiefs under "the standard code for ethics for chiefs in Sierra Leone." He would report a disaster to the District Office of the Ministry of Local Government, copied to the Office of National Security. Health issues would be reported to zonal health coordinators before reaching the DHMT. The Council of Paramount Chiefs is also another route to communicate health issues to the central government (interview, Foday Kamara, May 24, 2021). The advantage of the chief as a rapporteur for such threats is that he or she is more closely aware of any unusual developments than a touring official based in a provincial town.

Both the Paramount Chief of Jawei chiefdom and the section chief of the Koindu section in Kissy Teng chiefdom witnessed the first eruption of Ebola cases, and took leading roles in local response. In Jawei, the wife and daughter of the Paramount

[3] Election is a pre-colonial practice (Alldridge, 1901, p. 245).

Chief were among the first victims of the disease. It is also the case that as a former dispenser, he had some prior information about Ebola and was in personal contact with a virologist at Kenema Government Hospital, who provided immediate practical advice over the phone.

Self-quarantining for 42 days after his wife and daughter died, the chief organized (through his open window!) local volunteers to undertake case finding, quarantine and burial, and fought off significant amounts of Ebola denialism from people who thought the disease was a politically motivated hoax. He won these battles because the measures he and his volunteer teams imposed started to reduce the incidence of cases.

Other chiefs, linked daily by cellphone, started to apply the same measures with the same results. The Kailahun council of chiefs then met in Mandu chiefdom in late July 2014 to review their achievements and to endorse a set of Ebola bye-laws for the district. These were then quickly adopted at national level also (Government of Sierra Leone, 2014).

The influence of a Paramount Chief reaches only so far. However, one chief told us that he was unable to persuade the elders of the powerful women's Bundu society to change corpse preparation practices. Their rituals were none of his business. It needed an interlocutor who was a member of the association to talk to the female elders. The elders were asked what they did for burial in the old days when smallpox was a hazard. They described practical ways in which they had protected themselves against infection, and the interlocutor suggested that similar adaptations of burial practices should be introduced to guard against infection risks from Ebola (Mokuwa, 2020). Since this respected the authority of the women elders, they found it possible to agree.

The general lesson from this story of local agency becomes clear; biosecurity changes require cooperation with local responders. Infection challenges need to be explained by trustworthy interlocutors, and community leaders need to engage to bring about desired effects. Essential principles need to be internalized. Workarounds have to be applied. And the people and their leaders have to be supported to come up with solutions to key risks. Little if any of this infection control can be done by command and coercion alone.

Challenges and Obstacles

Importantly, local response in the first phases of the epidemic worked in Kailahun because there was not as yet any larger-scale response within which these local improvisations had to be accommodated. First responders in Kailahun were working with the support of only local government and locally deployed security forces. They were obliged to think for themselves, and to experiment, and they learnt from experience what did and did not work. If things went wrong, their own communities bore the brunt.

From September 2014, a scaled-up international response provided a framework of epidemiological theory to guide Ebola control. Actions were now subject to rational design and not local experiment. Importantly, international responders could reinforce their aims with money and abundance of material. Chiefs and local volunteers had to fit in or step back. This presented some challenges for the effectiveness of the response.

Whereas early efforts at Ebola control had been hampered by lack of key resources—such as lack of basic information, transportation, personal protective equipment (PPE), and supplies of chlorine—later in-country responses were sometimes undermined or distracted by sheer abundance of resources thrown at the problem by a panic-stricken international community. Super-abundance triggered struggles to command resources, fed corruption, and at times exacerbated political rivalries (Walsh & Johnson, 2018).

International providers, however, took little time to assess local capacities or were slow to learn from community experience. As the epidemic overwhelmed Kenema, hospital doctors and nurses started to warn colleagues in other districts by phone that the disease did not manifest itself in Sierra Leone according to the WHO case definition (Richards et al., 2020). Bleeding was not a major symptom, for example. In fact, the disease was hard to recognize since it (at first) mimicked more common conditions (notably malaria and typhoid). But it took some time for the case definition to be amended.

Second, the significance of bush meat as a factor in transmission was grossly over-stated. Warnings against hunting and bush meat were pushed out for many months as a central element in what WHO termed its "messaging approach" even though evidence from genomics suggested human bodily contact was the single greatest risk factor (Richards, 2016, p. 25).

In fact, villagers in Kailahun, Kenema, and Bo districts had worked this out for themselves in the first stages of the epidemic. Families noted that infection followed members who had nursed or buried an Ebola victim and named the disease in Mende (the main language of the region) *bonda wote*, "family turn away." Yet it took many months for local observation to change official messaging on the disease.

Likewise, international responders saw local improvisation, such as the use of plastic bags and reversed raincoats to handle "wet" cases as desperation measures, to be replaced as quickly as possible by (for example) "proper" PPE. A more constructive approach might have been to treat these measures as positive indicators that infection processes were well understood, and to build on this local awareness and ingenuity to spread messages about transmission pathways. Better than nothing in an emergency, plastic bags were potentially significant ways people could conceptualize disease threats in terms of familiar everyday objects. By contrast, alien PPE "moonsuits" unintentionally terrorized local populations.[4]

[4] In a workshop at Njala in 2015, a women's society elder from Jawei chiefdom asked for a PPE "moonsuit." Her plan was to construct a "dancing devil" to teach children how it protected the wearer from infection.

Unintended Consequences

Failure to integrate emergent local and international understandings of the disease had some serious unintended consequences.

Perhaps the clearest instance is the bush meat fiasco. Messaging over Ebola and bush meat induced an unhelpful belief among those who lived nowhere near a forest, or never ate bush meat as a matter of religious principle, that they were protected. Fortunately, rural communities surveyed in December 2014 had begun to use their own observational common sense and responded to risks posed by human contact (Richards, 2016, p. 81).

Unintended consequences for infection control were also linked to local political conflict. The western extremity of Moyamba district is an instance. The area suffered a surprising late surge in cases, as the outbreak was easing elsewhere in the district, and international response was mobilized to deal with it. A group of Norwegian medical volunteers set up and ran a small ETC in Moyamba from December 2014 to February 2015. Survival rates, however, were disappointingly poor when results were much better elsewhere. Case fatality rates were reported at about 58%, in contrast to 23% being achieved at that time in an adjacent ETC at Kerrytown.

Since the Norwegian and local staff were both deemed highly competent the Moyamba anomaly requires explanation. Haaskjold et al. (2016) make a crucial connection: "higher CFR in Moyamba could partly be explained by a bias favoring selection of severe cases from some of the less accessible areas that rely extensively on traditional medicine; in such areas, milder cases would have been treated locally" (Haaskjold et al., 2016, p. 1541). The implication is that local treatment delayed admission to the ETC of patients who might have been saved if admitted more promptly.

A retrospective ethnographic case study strongly confirms these speculations by the Norwegian responders. Parker et al. (2019) and colleagues offer detailed documentation of quite extensive efforts to care for Ebola cases in one community in Ribbi chiefdom. Their paper does not explain, however, why this local care had been happening in the case study community but apparently not in neighboring communities with Ebola cases.

Unpublished field notes by one of the present authors (GAM) provide relevant clues. The village had been stripped of its section headquarter status, and a government health center had been located elsewhere. Informants claimed they were boycotting government health provision due to the reduced administrative status of their village. Records suggest this boycott was not actually very effective, if it was taking place at all. But the arrival of case finders from district headquarters may have provided an opportunity for embattled community leaders to exemplify their complaint in more dramatic terms.

The political problem was an enduring one, dating back to the colonial period, and resolution was still pending in 2018. Cooperation over Ebola might have been seen as endorsing the official point of view. If so, it would appear that the Norwegian responders had the misfortune to become unwittingly entangled in a long-running local political dispute, with perverse medical consequences.[5]

Quite what might have been done to avoid this unfortunate situation is not entirely obvious. The case admission forms for Ebola cases were hard to complete for patients in late-stage sickness, so the background of patients was often unclear (Haaskjold et al., 2016). If the ETC staff had more clearly known the origins of their patients, the problem might have been more clearly identified. Faced with similar challenges Nganyahun ETC in Kenema deployed liaison officers to build information on the social background of infected persons, and keep families better informed on cases (Richards et al., 2019). It would have been an advantage to have a pool of well-trained social science graduates from which to recruit such personnel; alas, Sierra Leone lacks training and capacity in relevant fields such as medical anthropology.

The third unintended consequence of Ebola response in Sierra Leone should also be mentioned. This was the banning of traditional herbalists, for fear their activities spread the disease. Exclusion of herbalists, however, may have unintentionally undermined efforts against Ebola by silencing a potentially persuasive group of public interlocutors.

In a meeting in Bo to discuss the results of a study of local response to Ebola, a leading herbalist argued as follows: the government and international responders prevented herbalists from practicing during the epidemic, but since these practitioners were more trusted by their clients than formal medical practitioners, might it not have been better to train herbalists in the rules of Ebola infection prevention, and deploy them as front-line responders against the disease? No satisfactory answer was forthcoming.

Ebola and Lessons Learned

What Worked/Did Not Work and Why Not?

Local responders contributed more, and more effectively, to Ebola control in Sierra Leone than widely recognized. A rough indicator of the effectiveness of Ebola response in Sierra Leone is the period of time that elapsed between the first and last cases in the main administrative districts of Sierra Leone. This varied (in provincial districts) from 90 days in Bo district to 280 days in Port Loko District (see Table 1 in

[5] Experience of the COVID-19 pandemic (not least in the United States, approaching a bitterly divisive presidential election in 2019) makes it clear that political factionalism has a major influence over whether people believe messages about infection threats or accept the need for measures such as quarantine and vaccination. It should also be added that the Norwegian-assisted ETC was a replacement for a notorious case handling facility in Moyamba with very poor survival rates (Richards et al., 2020). It is unclear if these disaffected villages saw the two Ebola treatment facilities as distinct.

Richards et al., 2020). By and large the earlier an outbreak was in the timeline of the epidemic, the sooner it was ended, thus providing some support for a claim that local response and international support combined relatively more effectively in earlier than in later stages of the epidemic.

It is important to ask why this was so. This was in part due to the scale of the international response. Coordination became a challenge in itself, as abundantly illustrated by the very valuable eyewitness account of Walsh and Johnson (2018). Top-down management was emphasized in order to keep control of a vast and daily ramifying operation, and this in turn restricted the space for local agency. The international response to the recent North Kivu Ebola outbreak repeated some of the same mistakes (Ebola Gbalo, 2019). British response to COVID-19 has similarly been strongly criticized for over-centralization, and marginalization of local public health expertise, translating into poor infection control and dangerous viral mutations (Thomas & Clyne, 2021).

A key take-home message, therefore, is that local knowledge is an extremely valuable commodity in management of epidemics and needs to be protected, especially in a crisis atmosphere where common sense and calm judgment tend to be at a premium.

Health systems need to be more carefully configured to avoid a rush of essential resources obliterating local knowledge and expertise. It also needs to be more clearly recognized that much of the local knowledge and expertise of crucial value in an epidemic is social rather than medical in nature. For instance, the medical skills of the Norwegian volunteers and their local associates were put at risk in Moyamba for lack of knowledge of the micro-political landscape of Ribbi chiefdom.

Generating, valorizing, and protecting bodies of epidemiologically useful social knowledge is a challenge, especially in circumstances such as Sierra Leone, where scientific research has long been marginalized, with social science at the tail end of the queue for disbursements from a tiny national science budget. To avoid marginalizing local response initiatives, much greater effort has to be invested in identifying, creating, and deploying knowledge of how social factors interact with and shape epidemic outcomes. This lesson carries over into the management of the COVID-19 pandemic (see the next section).

Implications for Future Preparedness/Response

Future preparedness requires a better appreciation of the part that local responders play in epidemic response, especially in addressing social and cultural aspects, something which in turn requires better preparation of those local responders, especially in terms of social science skills relevant to recognizing, analyzing, and interpreting the local behavioral shifts needed to reduce infection transmission. This should extend to assessing and mobilizing bodies of traditional medical practice. Social science is especially important in organizing knowledge frameworks for local response, including understanding informal systems of medical care. For example, it helps with the clarification of complex and often ambiguous terms such as "culture" and "trust" (Chap. 1, Fig. 1.1) the sorting out of dependent and independent variables, and the separation of contextual factors and causal mechanisms, prior to the proper testing of hypotheses using adequately sampled data sets. Medicine and epidemiology, currently largely biological and mathematical sciences, need to become social sciences as well.

Comparison with COVID-19

Sierra Leone is an especially interesting case since it allows comparison between response to Ebola and COVID-19. Having experienced Ebola, the government of Sierra Leone reacted quickly and hard to the first cases of COVID-19 detected at the end of March 2020. Advice on the airborne nature of virus spread, social distancing, and quarantine was prepared and disseminated through local media, mainly radio and TV. Local awareness of this new disease threat was high.

A lockdown was then imposed in April 2020. International travel was suspended. Inter-district local passenger travel was also halted, though freight continued to move. A government computerized pass system was introduced to allow essential movement for a limited number of key workers. Lockdown was too draconian to sustain for long but imposing it promptly appears to have usefully slowed the initial advance of the disease while other response measures were put in place.

With German cooperation, laboratories were set up to administer PCR tests for COVID-19. Initial rates of testing were at first low, so no clear picture emerged about the spread of the virus, but community testing later allowed basic infection levels to be assessed. Cases were held at a low level, and international travel recommenced in July, but only for those who could show a negative PCR test for SARS Cov-2.

The virus is now found throughout the country, but infections appear to be greatest in the capital, which is where most deaths have also occurred. Case levels remain low but follow the pulsing of the disease internationally. A small first wave peaked in August 2020 and a second wave (again of low amplitude) occurred in January 2021, apparently boosted by international diaspora travel over the Christmas holiday period.

Cases that test positive are quarantined in a government military hospital. Patients are fed and treated well and are provided with funds to return home when quarantine is complete. Quarantine is highly unpopular, however. In part, this is because the disease is often mild or even asymptomatic, and patients simply do not believe they are ill. Quarantine is seen as arbitrary punishment, and a sign of authoritarian overreach, especially by those disinclined to vote for the current government.

Some initial assessments of local perceptions of the disease suggested that it was feared as much or more than Ebola. An experimental game (Kamara et al., 2020) was played in two villages in central Sierra Leone in April 2020, after the presence of the disease in Sierra Leone had been confirmed but before any cases had reached these villages.

One village had successfully resisted Ebola infection, the other had experienced a severe outbreak resulting in many deaths. Players were asked to assess two kinds of infections—one with low risk of infection and high risk of death (similar to Ebola) and the other with high risk of infection but low risk of death (similar to COVID-19). Neither disease profile was identified, though players quickly spotted the Ebola-type profile, and assumed the other must have been COVID-19.

Surprisingly, in both the villages, a majority of players showed most concern for the COVID-19 profile. We represented the risks associated with both diseases via heaps of stones. A significant number of players (~20%) spotted that the combined probability of infection and death was the same in both the cases. The rationale of those preferring the Ebola profile was that this was a disease they understood. Based on experience, they had confidence it could be avoided by applying sanitary rules. The COVID-19 profile worried them more, given they had been told over the radio it was an airborne disease, with less predictable spread. Radio commentators implied the disease might be worse than Ebola.

Continued follow-up in one of the villages suggests that perspectives on COVID-19 have now begun to change. Lockdown hit villagers especially hard, since the Paramount Chief, having imposed an effective quarantine during Ebola (his chiefdom was one of only a small number in entire country without any Ebola cases) again applied strong regulations to restrict local movement of persons. Farmers, for example, were given the choice of whether to remain in the village or in their farms. The closure of the local open-air periodic market was also of serious concern. Traders could no longer buy or bring in goods due to the ban on inter-district movement. COVID-19 lockdown was more severe than any movement restrictions in place during Ebola, and once the first cases were reported—many with mild symptoms—people began to wonder what purpose the restrictions served.

Although rules were relaxed from June 2020 much damage was done in the 2 months of strict lockdown. Some traders reported an entire loss of their trading capital. Farmers had been inactive at a key period in the planting season and now anticipated severe food shortages in coming months.

Village Health Workers (VHWs) had their contracts suspended in January, for lack of funding, shortly before the COVID-19 emergency was declared. These VHWs are the bottom level of healthcare provision of the Ministry of Health and Sanitation. They are permanent residents of their villages who have undertaken training in a basic set of health care modules, and as a result have enough knowledge to diagnose common illnesses. They prescribe basic drugs for diseases such as malaria and report on disease outbreaks. Complex cases are referred to chiefdom or district health centers.

VHWs we have interviewed have a good awareness of COVID-19 but have not yet seen any actual cases. This lack of visibility poses a problem for their clients, some of whom now doubt whether the disease is real, since symptoms are easily confused with other common diseases. Unwittingly, WHO added to this problem by suggesting that COVID-19 will become an endemic disease. To some villagers, this implied that it is something to be endured rather than prevented. Ebola proved to be eminently preventable. COVID-19 is much less certainly preventable, and this represents a big perceptual difference in local minds. If it cannot be prevented, why bother with the rules is the implied question.

VHWs also report that some of their patients entertain doubts about the need for vaccination for COVID-19, fed by anti-vaccination propaganda, much of which is circulated by diaspora relatives, and reaches remote villages by cellphone connections. VHWs themselves appear to believe the disease exists, is spread through breathing, and is thus more difficult to detect and control than Ebola.

In short, clear differences have now opened up between Ebola and COVID-19. Ebola can be readily prevented by avoidance of high-risk body contact, such as washing corpses without proper protection. COVID-19 is "in the air" and much more difficult to guard against. Prevention is also more of a puzzle than for Ebola.

The concept of social distancing is widely known in Sierra Leone but not well-understood. In part, this is because it is hard to explain since it combines two otherwise distinct elements—physical distance and frequency of interaction. Town dwellers, in particular, think crowding and intense interaction are unavoidable parts of urban life.

The value of mask wearing as a protection against airborne infection is often appreciated, though the cost of acquiring such protection deters many people. In two surveys contrasting attitudes to mask wearing in town and village, rural farmers showed a much higher awareness than urban petty traders that mask wearing protected others as much or more than the wearer. An explanation is that farmers live a cooperative life and are used to think about how to benefit the group, while urban petty traders are more competitive and think first in terms of individual advantage.

Vaccination will play a major part in bringing the COVID-19 pandemic under control. At present, much concern is rightly directed at vaccine logistics and how to escape the vaccine nationalism through which a number of countries (for reasons of domestic politics) think in terms of protecting their own populations first and foremost. Vaccine nationalism risks undermining the strategic moves needed to limit infection overall. Political grasp of the global meaning of the word pandemic is emerging only slowly (Richards & Cohen, 2021).

The other great worry is whether widespread vaccine skepticism will undermine global efforts at pandemic control. Small surveys in Bo and Kenema (major provincial towns) and our two rural case study villages provide some initial insight into this. They suggest that the purpose of vaccination is widely understood, and clearly differentiated from certain somewhat similar local practices of injecting herbal remedies under the skin. Informants recall childhood vaccination against preventable diseases, including measles and polio.

Urban informants are more likely to repeat anti-vaccination propaganda, to which they have been exposed via social media. Some informants were clearly worried about what they saw as the politicized nature of international vaccination efforts—that different vaccines are being launched by countries with competing agendas in Africa, notably China and the United States. They wonder whether this will have consequences for those who take the vaccinations. Rural informants are more likely to state they will take vaccination against COVID-19 provided the government mandates it.

Conclusion: On Pandemic Preparedness

In Ebola-impacted Sierra Leone, the willingness by government to take prompt and draconian action against the virus seems to have helped limit the spread of pandemic COVID-19, even at the cost of some social and economic dislocation. Lessons carried over from the Ebola experience included the importance of quarantine and of instituting effective systems of tracking, tracing and isolating disease contacts. The need to provide those quarantined with livelihood support if they were to remain in isolation was also a lesson well learnt, as was the importance of providing clear and honest information about the spread of cases.

It is worth noting that Liberia and Sierra Leone—the two countries worst affected by Ebola in 2014–2015—have (within West African region) two of the lowest rates of spread of COVID-19 to date. It is important to recognize, however, that COVID-19 is not Ebola and that engagement of local responders with communities, while as important for COVID-19 as for Ebola, is taking a different form.

In Sierra Leone, the family-based care and burial-specific signals of Ebola spread were made clear to all through careful observation and reporting backed up by effective testing, and some timely genomics (Richards et al., 2020). Some countries have shown that a similar approach can pay dividends for COVID-19 as well (Eichler et al., 2021), but the technical challenges are greater (especially for testing and genomic tracking) and countries such as Sierra Leone, with a weak infrastructural base for science, will have to invest heavily in relevant skills, including both laboratory capacity and social science.

COVID-19 spreads more by stealth, and this has begun to cause doubt among many about whether the disease is as serious as claimed, or indeed whether it exists at all. Village Health workers, as rural first responders, seem to be well-informed about COVID-19 and are potentially effective interlocutors in helping communities understand the differences between Ebola and COVID-19, but it is a point of concern that their continued employment is currently under threat.

At a more general level, some major differences between community response to Ebola and COVID-19 in Sierra Leone are now becoming clear. Initial data from both observation and interviews suggest that politically inspired doubts (apparent in Ebola in some chronically contested localities, but for the most part swept away later by a clear signal from the disease) are much more likely to accompany COVID-19. We can expect political disagreement to play a much more important part in shaping local infection response to COVID-19, which appears, worldwide, to flourish in places with the deepest political divisions. Acceptance of guidance concerning protective action will therefore depend heavily on general trust in formal institutions of government and their capacity to foster health across all groups and classes. The openness, competence, inclusiveness and cooperativeness of responders, whether local or international, will be crucial factors in ensuring compliance with health regulations and acceptance of vaccines.

Acknowledgments This chapter draws data from two research projects. Financial support for the Ebola Gbalo project and PPP (Pandemic Preparedness research project) is gratefully acknowledged from the UK Medical Research Council and the Wellcome Trust. Ebola Gbalo: MRC Grant MR/N015754/—title: *Building resilient health systems: lessons from international, national and local emergency responses to the Ebola epidemic in Sierra Leone*. PPP: Wellcome Trust (212536/Z/18/Z) Collaborative Award, *Pandemic preparedness: local and global concepts and practices in tackling disease threats in Africa*.

The authors would also like to thank Musa Kallon, Paramount Chief of Jawei Chiefdom, and Fayia Sundifu Brima Sovula IV, Paramount Chief of Kamajei Chiefdom, for the information provided.

References

Alldridge, T. J. (1901). *The Sherbro and its hinterland*. Macmillan.

Ebola Gbalo Research Team. (2019). Responding to the Ebola virus disease outbreak in DR Congo: When will we learn from Sierra Leone? *The Lancet, 393*(10191), 2647–2650.

Eichler, N., Thornley, C., Swadi, T., Devine, T., McElnay, C., Sherwood, J., et al. (2021). Transmission of severe acute respiratory syndrome coronavirus 2 during border quarantine and air travel, New Zealand (Aotearoa). *Emerging Infectious Diseases, 27*(5), 1274–1278. https://doi.org/10.3201/eid2705.210514

Government of Sierra Leone (GoSL). (2014). *Byelaws for all chiefdoms in Sierra Leone: Byelaws for the prevention of Ebola and other diseases, approved by Parliament on Friday 8th August 2014 under Section 29 of the Constitution of Sierra Leone Act No. 6 of 1991*. Freetown.

Haaskjold, Y. L., et al. (2016). Clinical features of and risk factors for fatal Ebola Virus Disease, Moyamba District, Sierra Leone, December 2014-February 2015. *Emerging Infectious Diseases, 22*(9), 1537–1544. https://doi.org/10.3201/eid2209.151621

Kamara, F. M., Mokuwa, E. Y., & Richards, P. (2020). How villagers in central Sierra Leone understand infection risks under threat of COVID-19. *PLoS One, 15*(6), e0235108. https://doi.org/10.1371/journal.pone.0235108

Lamontagne, F., et al. (2014). Doing today's work superbly well: Treating Ebola with current tools. *The New England Journal of Medicine, 371*, 1565–1566. https://doi.org/10.1056/NEJMp1411310

Mokuwa, E. Y. (2020). *Epidemics and community conflicts: The value of indigenous institutions in addressing development shocks in rural Sierra Leone*. PhD thesis, Wageningen University. https://doi.org/10.18174/533070

Mokuwa, E. Y., & Maat, H. (2020). Rural populations exposed to Ebola virus disease respond positively to localised case handling: Evidence from Sierra Leone. *PLoS Neglected Tropical Diseases, 14*(1), e0007666. https://doi.org/10.1371/journal.pntd.0007666. PMID: 31961858.

Parker, M., Hanson, T. M., Vandi, A., Babawo, L. S., & Allen, T. (2019). Ebola and public authority: Saving loved ones in Sierra Leone. *Medical Anthropology, 38*(5), 440–454. https://doi.org/10.1080/01459740.2019.1609472

Richards, P. (2016). *Ebola: How a people's science helped end an epidemic*. Zed Books.

Richards, P., Amara, J., Ferme, M. C., Kamara, P., Mokuwa, E., Sheriff, A. I., et al. (2015). Social pathways for Ebola virus disease in rural Sierra Leone, and some implications for containment. *PLoS Neglected Tropical Diseases, 9*(4), e0003567. https://doi.org/10.1371/journal.pntd.0003567

Richards, P., & Cohen, D. B. (2021, March 4). Africa and COVID-19: Why we need pandemic-scale political thinking. *African arguments* blog series.
Richards, P., Mokuwa, E., Welmers, P., Maat, H., & Beisel, U. (2019). Trust, and distrust, of Ebola treatment centers: A case-study from Sierra Leone. *PLoS One, 14*(12), e0224511. https://doi.org/10.1371/journal.pone.0224511. PMID: 31790420.
Richards, P., Mokuwa, G. A., Vandi, A., Mayhew, S. H., & Ebola Gbalo Research Team. (2020). Re-analysing Ebola spread in Sierra Leone: The importance of local social dynamics. *PLoS One, 15*(11), e0234823. https://doi.org/10.1371/journal.pone.0234823
Thomas, A., & Clyne, R. (2021). *Responses to shocks: 10 lessons for government*. Institute for Government.
Walsh, S., & Johnson, O. (2018). *Getting to zero: A doctor and a diplomat on the Ebola frontline*. Zed Books.
WHO. (2014). *Protocol on safe and dignified burial*. Freetown.

Chapter 7
The Invisible Threat: Communicating Risk and Engaging Communities to Respond to Zika

Julie Gerdes and Arianna Serino

Contents

Setting the Context

The U.S. Government was a major contributor to the Zika response in the Americas, mounting a $366.5 M direct effort that included social and behavior change, as well as community engagement, vector control, and health service delivery components. This chapter will focus on examples and lessons learned from the U.S. Government's (USG) international Zika response in Latin America and the Caribbean between 2016 and 2019.[1] Specifically, we focus on five themes that emerged from the Zika response: (1) the invisible threat of Zika; (2) the role of stakeholder coordination;

[1] The U.S. Government was the largest single donor to the Zika response in the Americas. It developed a multi-country implementation strategy that focused on countries with the greatest need for support and on existing bilateral relations with the U.S. that could be leveraged to work quickly. Because the U.S. Government's response was limited in geographic scope, our examples will focus on countries that implemented Zika response efforts with U.S. taxpayer funds, which notably excludes Brazil. Both the coauthors were employed full time to work on this response.

J. Gerdes (✉)
Department of English, Virginia Polytechnic Institute and State University, Blacksburg, VA, USA
e-mail: jgerdes@vt.edu

A. Serino
Behavior Change and Community Health Advisor, Washington, DC, USA

E. Manoncourt et al. (eds.), *Communication and Community Engagement in Disease Outbreaks*, https://doi.org/10.1007/978-3-030-92296-2_7

(3) participatory design of and collective community action in the face of urgent infectious disease programming; (4) the unintentional reification and/or reversal of gender and family support norms in Latin America and the Caribbean in Zika prevention messaging; and (5) opportunities for practices that advance the rights of children with disability promoted by social inclusion policies in the region. First, we reflect on challenges and opportunities during Zika programming, elucidating these issues with program examples, then we suggest lessons learned around these thematic areas for future social and behavior change programs responding to complex infectious disease threats.

Background

Serologists first identified the Zika virus in rhesus monkeys in the Zika forest of Uganda in 1947 (Dick et al., 1952). In 1948, the virus was found in an *Aedes africanus* mosquito, and in 1952, the first cases were identified in humans in Uganda and Tanzania (Dick, 1952; Smithburn, 1952). For many years, studies of the Zika virus focused exclusively on serology, isolating, and tracing the prevalence of the virus from Africa to Asia in both humans and mosquitoes and classifying the virus as mild and sporadic (Kindhauser et al., 2016). As a neglected tropical disease (NTD), Zika stayed largely under the radar in public health circles until an outbreak in Micronesia in 2007–2008 led to household epidemiological surveys, lab diagnostics studies, and a concentrated entomological investigation (Duffy et al., 2009; Lanciotti et al., 2008). This early Zika outbreak was downplayed among public health authorities, who had determined that symptoms of the virus were mild and associated with dengue (CDC, 2007; FSM Information Services, 2007).

In 2015, Zika exploded onto the global radar when clusters of fetal microcephaly—a condition in which a child is born with an abnormally small brain and head, leading to developmental delays—were reported among babies of women who had presented with mild rash and/or fever during their pregnancy. As the Brazilian surveillance system picked up an outbreak of the mosquito-borne Zika virus, clinicians in the outbreak area of Northeastern Brazil began sharing reports of increased microcephaly cases. It is now suspected that the previously mild virus mutated and that the mutation led to increased infectivity as well as the association with fetal microcephaly (Yuan et al., 2017; Rossi et al., 2018; Cugola et al., 2016). By February 2016, the outbreak had gained the international media spotlight, and the World Health Organization declared that the clusters of neurological disorders and neonatal malformations associated with Zika virus infection was a Public Health Emergency of International Concern (PHEIC).

This declaration triggered a landslide of additional funding and attention. One study on news coverage around public health authority announcements in January-February 2016, when a series of announcements that reported on the emergency state of Zika outbreaks in the Americas, demonstrates that both mass media and social media coverage of Zika in the United States, Guatemala, and Brazil experienced an "ephemeral peak" during the time of these announcements (Southwell et al., 2016). This media attention was exacerbated by the location of the upcoming summer Olympics in Brazil. In February 2016, scientists had established a link between Zika infection in pregnancy and microcephaly and confirmed that the virus could be transmitted sexually as well as from mosquitoes (vector transmission), but little more was known about the nature and effects of the virus. Stakeholder public health organizations developed risk communication materials for the Americas that were aimed at preventing mosquito breeding sites and protecting pregnant women from mosquito bites. These informational materials largely piggybacked and reinforced dengue and chikungunya messaging from recent years of those arbovirus outbreaks throughout the Americas.

Much has been learned about the virus since it leapt to front pages in 2015. We have learned that the virus is transmitted through three forms: (1) vector (primarily the *Aedes aegypti* mosquito) transmission, (2) vertical (mother-to-child) transmission, which can occur through the placenta at any time during pregnancy but is more likely during the first trimester, and (3) sexual transmission (female-to-male, male-to-female, male-to-male, and potentially, although undocumented, female-to-female). Congenital Zika syndrome (CZS) has replaced the more general label of "microcephaly" to more specifically and accurately describe the range of effects of in-utero Zika virus infection on a baby's physical and/or neurological development. Babies born with CZS may demonstrate traits similar to traditional microcephaly, but the syndrome also encompasses a number of other neuro-physical or developmental issues that can initiate months after birth. Zika can also lead to Guillain–Barre syndrome (GBS) in adults.

"Complexity" does not cover the enormous hurdles that behavior change scientists and practitioners were faced with in responding to Zika. On the one hand, the virus was not particularly fatal (although we suspect that more severe cases led to undetected miscarriages), and infection was asymptomatic in 80% of patients and mild in most others. However, there were major personal, social, and economic impacts of a potential generation of children in need of structural support and changes in health, educational, and community systems for a mosquito-borne virus that was becoming endemic. On top of that, the outbreaks caused national-level economic impacts on tourism that challenged communication efforts, and it exacerbated existing economic and health inequities caused by differences in access to lab testing and specialized care. Between risk perception, gender norms around prenatal care, and the multiple modes of transmission (each with its own set of recommended behaviors), behavioral aspects of responding to Zika was an incredibly complex puzzle of overlapping pieces at individual, community, and national levels.

In March 2016, the WHO published a Zika Knowledge, Attitudes, and Practices (KAP) resource pack developed for governments and response partners to adapt locally. This tool was deployed through the Pan American Health Organization (PAHO) "as a way to rapidly obtain valuable and insightful information in order to tailor interventions to better address people's needs at community level" (World Health Organization, 2016). Organizations implementing community engagement interventions used this tool in part as a response to the appetite for examining the local contexts of communities in the context of infectious disease outbreaks, which had been identified as a gap in the Ebola response. Intended to support the identification of key areas to further investigate, in practice, the tool served as a shared methodological framework for developing baselines and comparing routine progress across countries and sub-national communities.

The U.S. Government Response

By April, the U.S. Agency for International Development (USAID) was funding the U.S. Centers for Disease Control and Prevention (CDC), Johns Hopkins University Center for Communication Programs, and a number of other organizations to work on risk communication, knowledge management, and social and behavior change communication activities. Sub-regional, national, and local government entities, as well as PAHO, the European Union, and other global health and local nonprofit organizations had also been contributing to short-term, emergency response activities for vector control and risk communication. In September 2016, U.S. Congress approved $1.1 billion in funding for Zika response efforts, which kicked off a flurry of research and response activities across the United States and throughout Latin America and the Caribbean.

In acknowledgment of strong existing national programs and in an effort to improve the sustainability of time-limited programmatic funding, USG programs did not build vertical structures but rather plugged into existing infrastructure. For instance, in Haiti, the government was already working on mapping mosquito hot spots through the Program National de la Contrôle de la Malaria (PNCM; or *National Malaria Control Program* in French), and USG programming complemented this work by importing larvicide and training vector control technicians to apply the product in those hot spots. In terms of SBC, national governments and local media outlets had been warning citizens of Zika and promoting prevention strategies well before the U.S. Congress approved of funding. When new programs mobilized, they started with rapid assessment and stakeholder mapping before becoming involved in developing routine working group spaces that included members of national communications teams and that worked on adapting the USG-funded regional tools like job aids for volunteers conducting home visits.

This USG programming was developed in 2016 as a regional response that spanned across Latin America and the Caribbean and included programming out of Washington and Panama City as well as bilateral activities. The program focused on two pillars of vector control and health service delivery, to include maternal and child as well as family planning health systems. Within both pillars, community engagement and behavior change were emphasized, from community environmental clean-up campaigns to the formation of mothers' groups for those whose children were affected by Zika virus infection. High-level funding decisions are always political first, often well-intentioned second, and equitable last. Such was the course for the Zika response in the Americas, which saw several successes in transnational coordination but, due to the design of the response into relatively siloed technical pillars, missed opportunities to formally bring providers and vector control technicians into the behavior change fold, instead primarily focusing on mass media campaigns, interpersonal community engagement techniques, and building capacity for national communications strategies. Provider behavior change was framed within the scope of counseling guidelines, and vector control workers often implemented health promotion activities through the education component of their household visits. These two areas are largely outside of the scope of the current chapter, which will focus on social and behavior change communication work at the community level, on national communications strategies within affected Ministries of Health, and on general public guidelines and recommendations for Zika prevention and care.

Over the course of 3 years of implementation, community networks bound together to map communities, educate school children, and turn the dial on local vector control policies. However, the overreliance on quantitative surveys with large sample sizes and the need for validation in the face of evolving science, as well as the inherent complexity of Zika, missed the opportunity to engage deeply in what meaningful and large-scale ethnographic inquiry and locally informed solutions to mosquito control and early child development needs.

Reflection

As outlined in Chap. 1, elements of risk communication and community engagement (RCCE) in public health emergencies, from human rights to trust to culture, are organically linked to the point that addressing them as separate issues would disingenuously rupture a holistic view of the response. The Zika RCCE response was no different. While separate pillars worked on mosquito control and social inclusion of children with disabilities, these pillars intersected and overlapped in practice. For instance, clinicians counseled women who experienced gender-based violence to prevent mosquito bites during family planning sessions, and vector control technicians promoted community responsibility and incentivized community care during their household visits, often in neighborhoods experiencing gang violence or rapid emigration. Despite differences in functions and expertise, the complexity of Zika's disease dynamics and implications on a span of related social issues blurred traditional lines of responsibility, pulling all stakeholders into a role in promoting human rights, building trust, and considering culture at the core of their activities.

Zika was complex in many ways: there are still many scientific unknowns, in part because of the lifetime effects of congenital Zika syndrome; there are multiple transmission routes, and the origins of disease are impossible to distinguish outside of the lab; it circulated alongside other arboviruses; it caused a variety of issues including and in addition to microcephaly; and the intense concern for unborn life even led the Pope to okay the use of birth control pills in traditionally Catholic Latin American countries. These complex issues span those of biomedicine, entomology, culture, and rights and inclusion, and they came to fore in diverse ways across different country contexts.

The efforts of trying to control mosquitoes and sexual and reproductive lives while the world got a grip on defining this virus were monumental. Nevertheless, communities in Latin America where the USG response was implemented used a number of localized approaches to engage youth in prevention measures, to monitor mosquito breeding sites within their control, to directly support local government leaders with entomological data, and to mitigate rumors in order to get the word out on the threat of Zika. Moreover, women with children with congenital Zika syndrome forms networks and lasting bonds of practical and emotional support, and dedicated healthcare workers found creative ways to transform spaces into pediatric physical therapy units. As with many infectious disease outbreaks, response heroes emerged at the community level.

The Invisible Threat of Zika

As a largely asymptomatic disease that primarily affected unborn children months after infection, Zika virus carried a very low risk perception. The lag in time between being infected with the virus, in most cases without any symptoms, and seeing its potential negative impacts in the form of a child being born with congenital anomalies, made it challenging for individuals to perceive and stay alert to the threat. In addition to this, the relatively low incidence of congenital Zika syndrome in any one given community made the disease intangible to many community members. This posed not only a challenge for messaging to target populations of pregnant women and their families who might be affected by Zika infection but also for behavior adoption in their larger communities.

Because slowing the transmission of Zika required both individual and community adoption of new behaviors, low risk perception was a significant hurdle to behavior change responders for the duration of Zika outbreaks. Eighty percent of Zika cases were asymptomatic, and the other 20% generally had very mild symptoms that overlapped in some aspects with dengue or chikungunya infection. In fact, coming on the heels of dengue and chikungunya outbreaks in most affected geographies, Zika was regarded as relatively benign. Four serotypes of dengue fever have been plaguing the American tropics since the region re-emerged out of an era of *Aedes* eradication in the 1980s. Isolated outbreaks eventually erupted into regional epidemics by 2010, when over 1.7 million cases were reported (Dick et al., 2012). According to PAHO reports (2020), there were over 2.4 million cases in 2015, when nearly 1400 people died of dengue and over 3.1 million dengue cases in 2019 (although it has become less deadly). Severe dengue incidence coupled with chikungunya, which had emerged in the Americas in 2013 and led to over a million cases in a year (Yactayo et al., 2016), led to some confusion over concomitant circulation of yet another arbovirus in the region. Chikungunya, however, was highly symptomatic, and patients would often cringe when remembering joint pain that accompanied their infection as entire populations of Caribbean islands were seemingly infected.

Zika virus outbreaks also occurred alongside yellow fever outbreaks in Brazil in 2016–2018 and rare-strain Mayaro virus outbreaks in Haiti and Brazil. The number of circulating threats became a lot for health departments, much less patients, to prioritize. Nevertheless, the long-term impact of Zika's effects on the next generation continued to garner its attention within the international community and among health departments in the region. Images of unborn children with severe microcephaly flooded communications avenues, urging expecting parents to wear condoms and avoid mosquitoes. Caribbean countries—a subregion in which transmission occurred later than in South and Central America—had been waiting with bated breath in anticipation of massive crippling effects on its small neonatal and child health systems. As the epidemic got downgraded from a PHEIC in November 2016, and countries outside of Brazil and Colombia were not seeing huge populations of congenital Zika syndrome characterized by severe microcephaly, fear waned and took risk perception with it.

Around the same time, the scientific community began developing findings on the wide range of consequences of congenital Zika syndrome on developing children. Cohort studies found that many children born to women with Zika infection were affected by developmental delays that either did not appear or did not fully manifest until after birth (Burger-Calderon et al., 2020; Van der Linden et al., 2016; Bhatnagar et al., 2017). Furthermore, poor neonatal outcomes such as central nervous system impairment were found to worsen as children born with Zika age, leading to severe motor impairment and affected children to fall exponentially behind in reaching developmental milestones, leading to need for increased advocacy and support (Satterfield-Nash et al., 2017). While pediatric healthcare workers were appropriately concerned and responsive to addressing these issues, many children affected by the first 2 years of the virus' circulation escaped surveillance by pediatric healthcare systems, in part because of public understandings of Zika as a threat only at or prior to the time of birth. Because the impact of early messaging about small head circumferences associated with severe microcephaly had penetrated the public conscience about Zika, it was difficult to retroactively inflict a more nuanced association among patients.

On top of the concurrent and recent felt arbovirus outbreaks, the asymptomatic nature of Zika virus infection in most adults, and the updates to science around congenital Zika syndrome, the role of tourism on many country's economies had a substantial impact on how countries elevated the disease's profile. A report by the United Nations Development Programme (2017) estimated a short-term cost of US$7–18 billion over 3 years, with most of the short-term costs attributed to international tourism revenue losses. This loss was estimated to reach $6.5 billion overall across Latin America and the Caribbean. In the Caribbean, these losses were expected to approach 1% of national GDPs in countries like Barbados and Saint Lucia and over 2% of the GDP in Aruba and the U.S. Virgin Islands. The World Bank calculated lost income from reduced international tourism to cost the region $10.5 billion over 3 years. In fact, in the first half alone, the U.S. Virgin Islands saw a loss of $250,000 in the first 6 months of 2016 due to travel cancellations, which is likely only a small portion of the impact during that time due to airlines offering free cancellations to Zika-affected countries (Qureshi, 2017, 2018, p. 140).

In response to Zika and other recent health concerns such as H1N1 and chikungunya, the Caribbean Public Health Agency (CARPHA) released a statement on its holistic approach to handling Zika and tourism, concluding "Don't let the mosquitos ruin your travel!" Instead, it urged behavioral practices to both prevent mosquito bites among individuals and to urge business to undertake vector control practices in and around guest lodging (Indar, 2016). The tension between public health guidance to avoid international travel and the economic dependence on travelers led to mixed perceptions of risk not only among local private sector stakeholders but also among populations from outside of high-risk areas who contemplated their own travel plans.

As a result of low-risk perception, the adoption of Zika prevention behavior was low. Material costs of some behaviors (such as using mosquito repellent) was high, and feasibility of other behaviors (like removing standing water and frequent scrubbing of water containers) was low, and without a high-risk perception, citizens were not motivated to overcome barriers to wholeheartedly adopt them.

Coordination of Stakeholders

Stakeholder coordination is a core concept sprinkled and promoted throughout international development discourse, particularly around the Global Health Security Agenda and disaster response (Kieny et al., 2016; Joshi et al., 2021). The idea is that during a time-sensitive, high-profile, and somewhat unpredictable event, concerns from all affected parties should be represented and addressed in forums that encourage consensus building and rapid decision-making. In the Zika response, coordination was central to successes in determining social and behavior change strategies, aligning Ministry of Health priorities with those of the U.S. Zika response objectives, and connecting relevant providers and specialists for quality infant care. Nevertheless, the siloed structure of the response and its mechanisms led to unnecessary challenges in infusing and streamlining social and behavior change best practices in clinical and vector control technical settings and in connecting community leaders with authority figures.

Early in the Zika response, an international working group on Zika social and behavior change began routinely meeting to discuss relevant studies, strategies, and topics of shared concern. This group of stakeholders from across the donor and nonprofit implementing community helped collectively digest scientific information about the disease as it emerged, coming to consensus on ways to incorporate or address new information. It also developed shared resources such as training and job ad materials for volunteers tasked with door-to-door education campaigns, and it encouraged stakeholders to share resources through the response's knowledge management website, the Zika Communication Network. The development and use of this site was one of many knowledge management successes that came out of Ebola lessons.

The international working group successes at donor headquarters was mirrored by several countries' Zika communications national working groups. By having local nonprofit stakeholders exchange information from international discussions with Ministry of Health counterparts, the parties were able to align objectives and build consensus around ways forward, determining what made sense in their national context and how to adapt materials to local settings. Moreover, these working groups established a flexible coordination system that could be stood up in future similar outbreak responses.

One activity that community engagement implementing organizations and UNICEF country offices successfully rolled out was stakeholder mapping. While UNICEF's priority was largely around mapping care and support specialists to link to clinical services needed by congenital Zika syndrome patients, community organizations mapped out networks of homes and businesses to engage in prevention activities within specific geographical areas. These maps enabled organizations to not only be systematic in their coverage and approach but also to guide purposeful coordination with local businesses and homeowners, improving collective community prevention and action against the spread of Zika.

Collaboration practices can generally be complicated and difficult when stakeholders are misaligned around priorities or theories of change. The U.S. Government Zika response, however, actively combatted issues by developing spaces for sharing and articulating clear program objectives. In fact, the coordinated nature of the Zika response was well-received by global health experts who have worked in the region for years, praising it as one of the least messy and most coordinated activities in memory. In large part, that can be attributed to the clear roles of each implementing organization within the overall structure of the response. At the same time, this approach challenged the full integration of social and behavior change science into technical areas of clinical service delivery and vector control. Namely, provider behavior change practices were either neglected in some settings or handled by clinical experts rather than behavior change experts, and household visits by vector control technicians were informed by principles of entomology but not intentionally informed by behavior change priorities. Over time, these organizations stepped outside of their siloes and collaborated, largely as a result of individual recommendations or program-wide meetings.

For instance, the Zika AIRS Project, or ZAP, led the U.S. Government response in international vector control implementation for Zika. In some countries, ZAP technicians helped train community volunteers on relevant entomology and vector control and monitoring practices so that they could collectively cover more ground in household visits. The Breakthrough-ACTION Project under Johns Hopkins Center for Communication Programs, an expert in social and behavior change, trained ZAP technicians on interpersonal communication, recognizing their potential impact by virtue of routine household visits.

Collective Community Action in Face of Urgent Infectious Diseases

Because like other emerging infectious diseases, there was no cure or prophylaxis for Zika infection, it required community and individual action for prevention. The task of eliminating common mosquitoes from tropical areas where people have been living for years alongside them was challenging in three ways: (1) material, (2) community responsibility and policing, and (3) shifting transmission perspectives.

First, successful entomological monitoring and control is expensive. It requires large teams of trained, often seasonal, technicians to cover entire neighborhoods and, in some cases, regions, on a weekly basis. While most countries affected by Zika maintained budgets for modest vector control support after years of dengue and chikungunya outbreaks, the widespread nature of infected *Aedes aegypti* stretched those budgets to unsustainable investments. One solution that communities developed, often with the support of established local non-profit organizations, was a shared responsibility model. In this approach, community leaders would organize environmental clean-up campaigns, educating their neighbors on the mosquito life cycle and on at-home prevention measures to encourage long-term, low-cost behavior change. In notable successes, community networks worked with local health authorities to monitor entomological data using low-tech "ovitraps," which allowed people to track trends in mosquito populations at their homes and businesses and connect them to official databases to help identify hot spots and thus target government expenditures.

The Zika outbreaks in the Americas came at a time when public health media campaigns had started shifting from displays of government action to appeals to personal responsibility. Although the idea of "healthy lifestyles" had taken hold in the late twentieth century, the idea that environmental health and infectious disease concerns would be considered part of a healthy lifestyle had not taken hold. In fact, most citizens referred to the government as the primary agent in vector control, from pointing to fumigation images in the paper or in their experiences as effective responses to criticizing the lack of fumigation or environmental clean-up efforts on the part of their governments. Vector-borne diseases had been plaguing the Americas for years, but the focus on unborn children shifted the focus from personal responsibility for one's own health to a focus on community health. By controlling the mosquitoes that carry Zika in their yards and community spaces, citizens were protecting their pregnant neighbors, a concept that raised the stakes in tight-knit communities.

A significant challenge of the Zika response which will be familiar to public health practitioners working on urgent threats is the need to balance the perception of urgency with that of participatory design. Often, when we think of community-led interventions, we are supportive in theory but fear the lengthy timeline that participatory design takes to do effectively. This was the case in the Zika response community engagement portfolio, which was developed in recognition of the need to listen and respond to community concerns in responding to public health threats.

In practice, however, one shortcoming of this activity was its overreliance on top-down and hyper-pragmatic technical approaches to vector control and prevention messaging. Projects were designed in offices and often at regional level for quick approval, so that implementation could start rapidly, which was well intended to reach audiences while Zika was circulating. Unfortunately, this rush eliminated a crucial participatory design processes with community members, including negotiation around the feasibility of proposed prevention behaviors. This led to tension between messages and cultural norms that could have otherwise been anticipated in design phases. It also prevented the formation of a critical feedback loop between the project implementers and the communities they served. This often meant that programs were not community owned, and thus rather than embracing personal responsibility to care for one's neighbors, citizens often commented that preventing Zika was the role of their government. We do not mean this as a blanket criticism of the organizations who were actively working with and listening to community members in their work across the portfolio. Rather, we aim to illuminate the structural and historic issue of program design processes that have been developed with a model of expertise that centers on theoretical and academic knowledge and de-centers community members' lived experiences.

Gender and Family Support Norms: Reification and Reversal

Gender

The Zika response confronted machismo culture. Health leaders urged male partners to become involved in the protection of their unborn children by attending counseling sessions with their pregnant partners and by using condoms throughout the course of the pregnancy. However, uptake of these suggestions was low, and even when condoms were distributed cost-free during prenatal visits, women were faced with the task of explaining the complex circulation of virus from mosquito to sexual fluid to fetus on their own. The implication, after years of the promotion of condoms in the face of multiple partners in response to HIV/AIDS work, was that by taking condoms home, women were suggesting infidelity—a risk that many were not willing to take, with women reportedly tossing them in trash bins just outside of clinics.

At the time of Zika outbreaks, family planning programs in the Americas had reached many milestones, at least in terms of awareness and uptake of short-acting contraceptive use (Fagan et al., 2017; de Leon et al., 2019; Bertrand et al., 2015). With large networks of public and private options for contraception and family planning counseling, the region was well positioned to include Zika information in existing systems. Given that there were strict anti-abortion laws in most affected countries, such counseling was informative and based on an ethics of sexual health and suggestions of delaying pregnancy during the time of the outbreaks by using protection or abstaining.

The work of changing societal norms to include male partners in pregnancy care would take years. While some male partners did become involved in pregnancy and beyond, structural barriers and existing norms, such as employers not allowing men to take time off work for antenatal care visits, continued to pose barriers. Many women whose babies would be affected by Zika brought their abuelas (grandmothers) to postnatal care sessions, highlighting the incidence of teenage pregnancies in areas with high Zika risk and incidence.

Zika response efforts initially and inadvertently also contributed to the existing burden of work for women in the household by promoting a range of household behaviors such as removing standing water and scrubbing water barrels to remove mosquito breeding sites. In an attempt to respond to the issue of reinforcing existing gender norms, mass media campaigns in the second half of the Zika response built on the masculine trope of family protector, idealized men appeared in public announcements, urging them to take care of their families with the slogan "cuida tu familia del Zika" by taking on prevention behaviors like removing standing water and keeping their houses "clean"—tasks that were traditionally assigned to women, as well as new behaviors like attending counseling sessions and wearing condoms during pregnancy. Nevertheless, much of the regional mass media campaign and the clinical guidelines were framed around the assumption and promotion of nuclear family structures.

The idea of protecting the baby became the fulcrum of Zika prevention arguments in mass media because risks to unborn babies is exactly what distinguished this disease from dengue and chikungunya. However, when aimed at an audience of male partners, the message left out a massive group of single mothers It also reified conservative and colonial gender and family norms, painting the picture of small families consisting of two cis-gendered heterosexual and monogamous parents, often with one-to-three children, conservative clothing, and urban jobs. While this may have resonated with a segment of the population, it did not necessarily paint a picture of reality or even romanticized dreams for many sexually active young urban and peri-urban people. In some campaigns, particularly those focused on community engagement around vector control, the central framework for promoting these behaviors shifted from the responsibility of the male partner to that of the entire community to care for its next generation of children being born.

This shift was largely successful, moving the behavior motivation from one of personal responsibility for a healthy lifestyle to community responsibility for community health and success. Over the 3 years, communities organized nearly 38,000 Zika events that included schools, local governments, and community organizations, and over 1500 affected communities developed their own plans to prevent and control Zika.

In some cases, such as northern Haiti, citizens were united by mural art competitions among neighboring communities that built social cohesion, knowledge, and a shared sense of responsibility. Similarly, school-based work was conceptualized as a way of making children "agents of change" within their own families. The idea was that young students would take home lessons about vector control from school and teach their parents to reduce breeding sites around the house. However, in

Jamaican and other Caribbean cultures, the turning over of authorities to school-aged children at home countered norms and was largely unsuccessful. Nevertheless, many schools built Zika clubs and formed their own communities of vector control agents within school yards. These clubs, with distributed responsibility built on a care for the (school) community, became a sustainable network of next-generation citizens educated in vector control. Ultimately, over 1000 schools in the region came out of the response with tools and methods to address arbovirus threats.

Family Structures

Community engagement activities in the Zika response often promoted the use of school-based activities wherein children were positioned as agents of change. The idea was that if children learned about the mosquito life cycle and vector control practices at school, then they would go home and educate the adults in their homes, which would spread awareness and uptake among communities. This approach had varying degrees of success. In Central America, organizations received awards for the success of school-based projects. Nevertheless, a study by Save the Children and the International Federation of Red Cross and Red Crescent Societies concluded, however, that across Latin America and the Caribbean, this model was not working to replicate messages as much as these projects had assumed (International Federation of Red Cross and Red Crescent Societies, 2017). In fact, Posada et al. (2018) found that "Zika education at school level was not seen as a way of reaching household members." "Agents of change are not replicating messages as much as we assume." It is probable that the theory of change around knowledge transfer from child to adult was based on the assumptions about family structures that were more routed in Catholicism's ideals of nuclear families than it was on actual family structures in the region.

For instance, children in Jamaica are beloved by their families, who use corporal punishment as a common means of helping children learn (Steely & Rohner, 2006; Smith & Mosby, 2003). Steely and Rohner (2006) cite studies out of the University of the West Indies, indicating that corporal punishment happens at every socioeconomic level. Largely because of the use of corporal punishment, the witnessing of violent aggression at home, and an emphasis on obedience to authority, the parenting style in Jamaica has been characterized as "authoritarian" (Samms-Vaughan et al., 2005; Smith & Moore, 2013). However, Burke et al. (2017) complicate the logic about parenting, finding that "Jamaican mothers engaged in and valued intimate social interactions with their children, which was characterized by positive mutuality, openness, emotionally significant feelings of relatedness, and mattering" (p. 8). They suggest that expression of pride and affection over a child's achievement may lead to closeness in child–parent relationships rather than a more western construct of intimacy that involves mutuality. With this lens, the assumption that a child's closeness to their family members will be leveraged to share information is misplaced. Perhaps because of the emphasis on child obedience, it could be seen as deviant for a child to be "teaching" their parent.

Public health practitioners often invoke family norms in their behavior change strategies in a number of ways. Another space where this occurred in Zika messaging was through appeals to male partners. The assumption was often that engaging men in prenatal counseling would lead to more informed practices around how and why their unborn child needed protection from the mosquito-borne disease. While this framing was very successful for cis-gendered heterosexual long-term partners, it excluded the more marginalized and vulnerable populations such as women who were pregnant by rape or gender-based violence or who had been abandoned by their reproductive partner. Often, women who had children with congenital Zika syndrome came to postnatal care appointments with their mother, grandmother, or another community member who supported them.

Members of non-normative and non-nuclear family structures have the right to protection from damaging infectious disease outbreaks. Understanding what is important to close family ties requires abandoning assumptions about those values, abstaining from judgment, and invoking deep listening exercises in the form of ethnographic qualitative and participatory research.

Pushing the Needle on the Rights of Children with Disability

As mothers and clinicians alike began to realize the full range of effects of congenital Zika syndrome, health systems began to map services needed to those that existed. Meanwhile, at the local level, non-profit organizations supported the development of mother networks that provided sounding boards, connection, and support to one another. These connections often led to longstanding relationships that included in-person meetings as well as regular WhatsApp message groups in which topics ranged from health-related exchanges to celebrating their children's achievements.

Congenital Zika syndrome also forced formal medical systems in the Americas to confront issues of rights to specialized healthcare and education systems to re-evaluate their level of inclusion of children with disabilities. Countries in Latin America led the way in ratifying the Convention on the Rights of Persons with Disabilities after its approval in 2006, signaling high levels of policy support for people living with disabilities in the region. However, socioeconomic inequality and social exclusion are high in Latin America, compounding problems of un- and under-employment and poverty for those living with disabilities (Angel-Cabo, 2015, p. 97). Despite these systemic inequities, there is a large social support for disability advocacy. Zika outbreaks increased awareness of gaps and inequities in social services for children with developmental delays and motor impairments. One positive unintended consequence of the outbreaks was the mobilization of additional resources from regional, national, and local levels that will benefit not only

Zika-affected children but all children born with congenital developmental problems, including microcephaly and a range of other disorders.

Advocacy for these resources came from all levels. In Guatemala, a team of healthcare workers who were treating patients with congenital Zika syndrome converted a space in their facility for physical therapy of all infants with microcephaly and similar challenges. In Paraguay, where the country followed it National Plan for Comprehensive Early Childhood Development (2011–2020), Zika programming supported implementation of the UNICEF Care for Child Development Model. Zika programs there not only created quality improvement teams in hospitals in the Capital, Central, and Alto Paraná regions but also helped establish 14 early stimulation rooms and 14 evaluation clinics that served over 560 children with early infant stimulation appointments and evaluated 2294 children for developmental delays (URC, 2020).

Across the region, quality improvement teams were developed under the Zika program to improve newborn screening for disabilities, pairing these efforts to psychosocial support to affected families, early infant stimulation activities, and neurodevelopment surveillance—efforts that aligned to regional commitments to social inclusion in the education sector and helped families with a holistic approach to caring for their children.

Conclusions

Lessons Learned and Implications

There are several takeaways from the Zika behavior change response in the Americas that will be useful for public health practitioners in a wide range of infectious disease and outbreak settings. While there is a great deal of work to be done on the advocacy front to ensure that persons affected by outbreaks, from survivors to long-haulers to family caregivers, are not forgotten, Zika magnified the need for the public health community to advocate for the social inclusion of people with disabilities, particularly in resource-constrained environments. That said, we hope to offer some pragmatic recommendations around practices that responders can implement in real time from the beginning of outbreak response implementation.

First, we will present Zika-specific lessons learned, and then we will reflect on broader implications for future outbreak responses.

Factors that make Zika unique to other disease outbreaks include:

- The disease is not fatal, so it is difficult to justify among high-level decision-makers the mobilization of resources for eradication over other public health priorities. Instead, responders were dealing with the introduction of a new disease threat that was likely to stick around.
- There are three unique transmission pathways: vector/mosquito, vertical, and sexual. Each requires attention on different behaviors that would typically be

siloed into separate technical subject areas but, in the case of trifold disease transmission, requires intense collaboration to avoid confusion and fatigue among target populations and their communities.

- Zika has a very targeted population of at-risk vulnerable people (unborn and infant children) who cannot speak or act for themselves.
- Zika did not overwhelm health systems or overload hospitals with new patients. Rather, it required intense changes to existing healthcare practices within reproductive, maternal, and child health systems of care.

There are countless lessons from Zika about overcoming and embracing complexity in social and behavior change programming during infectious disease outbreak responses. In this chapter, we have outlined five key areas of invisible disease threat, stakeholder coordination, collective community action, gender and family support norms, and the rights of children with disabilities. Below, we outline takeaways and recommendations for each of these areas.

Invisible Disease Threat

The low-risk perception of Zika that stemmed from its perceived distance and invisibility resulted in a lack of motivation to take preventative action. One finding from the response was that citizens were more likely to take action when Zika was framed under the umbrella of infant health. In fact, the second of two major regional mass media campaigns, developed by Population Services International and called "Mamá Segura, Bebé Seguro de Zika," focused directly on the health of unborn babies. Moving from animated graphics portraying multiple family members to photography depicting pregnant women, the campaign argued, "Tu Bebé lo Vale todo" (Your Baby Is Worth Everything). This shift was due to research demonstrating that the strongest motivator for adopting prevention measures among the most at-risk population, pregnant women and their partners, was the health of their unborn child. The emotional appeals of this approach matched the target population's priorities, and while this approach did not fully overturn low-risk perception issues (e.g., understanding of sexual transmission remained low even despite this campaign), it did increase motivation and concern for a threat that was otherwise unconvincing. We recommend that formative research in future infectious disease responses investigate motivators for adopting prevention behaviors early and design campaigns around rhetorically positioning said values and priorities at the center of messages.

Given how late this shift came in the response, national governments and public health stakeholders should incorporate preparedness plans that include rapid ethnographic analysis of existing perceptions around relevant topics. For instance, had Zika responders quickly analyzed the perceived threat and nuisance of mosquitoes in affected communities, perceptions of family structures, and emotional relations to newborn children, communication divisions would not have had to use trial and error to test messages. Ministries of Health would need to support this formative research and rapid analysis through pandemic preparedness planning initiatives that elevated communication and community engagement as central to infectious disease response rather than a supplement to other biomedical interventions. Understanding infectious disease through this volume's conceptual framework could lead to meaningful financial and human resource support for early investigation into community values and perceptions of cultural issues that are implicated by new threats, particularly when they are invisible.

Stakeholder Coordination

Two critical lessons around stakeholder coordination are: (1) integrated program design is important for coordinated behavior change efforts; and (2) programs should develop and commit to routine working groups or similar spaces for routine collaboration.

During the course of the multiyear Zika response, public health officials came to appreciate the role of behavior change work across all facets of the infectious disease ecosystem. While it had largely been considered a "cross-cutting" endeavor in theory, the work of social and behavior change communication in practice became relegated to health promotion offices in Ministries of Health, who were often understaffed, underfunded, and under pressure to develop quick-win mass media campaigns on the fly. Promoting community-based behavior change research and innovation among the highest levels of government was a priority of the USG response, and the success of emerging infectious disease programs moving forward will rest on the ability of governments to embrace local approaches. For instance, vector control technicians used simple yet effective motivating strategies to encourage regular household protection measures. In some countries like Honduras, technicians used a positive reinforcement system in the form of low-cost smiley stickers. When a technician visited a house on their route and found no positive containers (water storage containers that had *Aedes* pupae or larvae), the homeowner would receive a happy face sticker on their weekly chart. Upon receiving this reward, community members became so proud of their "clean" homes that their motivation and friendly neighborhood competition would lead them to adopting daily vector control behaviors.

Second, the success of coordination tables and regular working groups appeared in multiple evaluations of Zika program elements. These groups are common at the beginning of emergency government responses, but they have a tendency to disband after an early emergency phase has passed. The Zika program illuminated the benefits of ongoing support for working groups. One key element was ownership and management of these meetings; without a clear leader or leading organization to set the agenda and ensure that the appropriate people were invited, groups fell apart and collaboration broke down. This was uncommon in the response in part because the U.S. Government, as lead donor, generally had a representative manage meeting times and spaces in country and delegated the leadership of the SBC working group to an expert organization at the headquarters level.

Collective Community Action

Community needs were central, in theory, to the Zika response. In practice, we learned three key lessons: (1) social accountability needs to be emphasized and incentivized early; (2) behavior prioritization should include issues of feasibility within one's lived experiences; and (3) successful programs recruit and train personnel from within target or at-risk communities.

We have reviewed the exigence for consideration of social accountability beyond but including personal responsibility for prevention of disease. We find that considering this issue upfront is critical but difficult. Many communities have distrust in outside and, specifically, medical authorities for very valid reasons and yet need to understand information important to their own health and wellness and that of their families. Practitioners should seek to understand barriers to uptake of social accountability. In some cases, people were incentivized to practice vector control when efforts were part of a larger competition or when they were awarded recognition for their actions. In school settings, children learned about Zika and freed school grounds of *Aedes* breeding sites through fun afterschool activities and games. Meaningful incentives and public recognition often helped to build trust in healthy practices, reframing them under the umbrella of play rather than work and lessening tensions.

A challenge of the Zika response was the vast number of behaviors that were promoted during the initial outbreak period. Over 30 behaviors were found to be promoted among target populations in the response, mostly falling under the vector control umbrella and others related to sexual health and attending health services. Given the rich history of vector-borne disease in the region, promoted behaviors ranged from locally sourced solutions with limited evidence of effectiveness (e.g., burning lemongrass) to highly effective yet expensive behaviors (e.g., use of commercial mosquito repellent when outdoors, installing window screens, and running air conditioning). A key activity that behavior change scientists developed was a prioritization of key behaviors based on feasibility, effectiveness, and efficacy. The focus on feasibility brought people's lived experiences under direct consideration, elevating issues of personal finances, lifestyles, and experiences to a level alongside issues of efficacy and effectiveness.

Another key takeaway from the Zika response was that programs who recruited volunteers and paid employees from within the community experienced much more success with access and trust than those who mobilized specialists from other parts of the country. The importance of building local capacity from within at-risk communities is central to success in infectious disease responses, even if it requires more time upfront in training and developing personnel.

Gender and Family Support Norms

While gender was a key consideration of the Zika response from the beginning, women were initially and inadvertently centered as both vulnerable to the effects of Zika and responsible for preventing that risk. Issues of gender-based violence were lamented, but programs were not intentionally designed around issues of gender-based violence, gendered and age-based family norms around household responsibilities, and even less around underrepresented or marginalized family structures of LGBTQ+ couples and single-parent households. During the response, the effects of this unintentional norming of hetero nuclear family structures became apparent in low prevention behavior uptake around condom use, low degrees of knowledge transfer between children and their adult supervisors in some contexts, and, to a degree, increases in unbalanced and gendered household responsibilities default assigned to women for vector control.

In the future, responses to outbreaks—arbovirus and otherwise—should consider gender in all aspects of design. Reflecting on assumptions about gender that are baked into theories of change for any intervention are good practice in public health but can be overlooked in the urgency of an outbreak response. Moving forward, this issue should be framed within the realm of effectiveness, considering how misogynistic practices, even unintentional, contribute not only to poor equity but also to low behavior uptake. Moreover, monitoring efforts should aim to interrogate gender beyond basic indicator demarcation. In other words, analyzing key SBC performance indicator metrics by gender is a helpful tool for initiating thoughts and identifying issues for further inquiry, but it is not enough. Anticipating that unintended consequences are possible, project teams should have a plan for monitoring and correcting issues of added burden on the part of female-identifying stakeholders in order to support more equitable and more effective practices.

Rights of Children with Disabilities

A positive consequence of the Zika response was that it supported practices that contributed to policy movements to advocate for the rights of infants and children with disabilities and the mainstreaming of disability work across a range of different health programs. Although the response initially focused on prevention, education, and essentially containment of the virus through vector control and through prenatal and family planning services, it ultimately shifted to include care and support mechanisms for families affected by congenital Zika syndrome. Although these efforts focused on the US Congressional mandate of Zika-specific work, they should have lasting positive impacts on all children born with microcephaly and similar challenges. In order for these benefits to be maximized, they need to be systemic. When an outbreak illuminates existing gaps in systems such as supply chain bottlenecks in the case of Ebola or child development services in the case of Zika, responders should design programs that support countries' existing policy platforms and not try to work in a vertical fashion.

Final Words

We still do not have a vaccine for the Zika virus. Whether one will be fully developed is unclear, but what is clear is that after the initial outbreaks, the region experienced Zika fatigue. Many island countries and lower elevation areas of Central America approached herd immunity. Others had to shift focus to dengue outbreaks in 2018–2019, and to COVID-19 in 2020. In this context, behavior adaptation to protect pregnant women continues to be the best response action if we are to see clusters of congenital Zika syndrome re-emerge. What else is clear is that while Zika is largely "over" for the vast majority of people in the Americas, its effects continue to be felt among the caregivers of children with congenital Zika syndrome. These children have a right to education, to future work, and to healthcare access free of discrimination. While national systems continue to work toward supporting diverse needs of diverse children, individuals and communities will undoubtedly lead the way as role models for effective and compassionate care.

Zika taught us that public health practitioners can better prepare for outbreaks by embracing the communication and engagement centered conceptual framework in their preparedness and early response plans. By acknowledging the layered and intersecting messiness of diseases as they move through, illuminate, and show disregard for issues of human rights and culture, communications officials as well as networked actors from vector control technicians to pediatric care specialists (in the case of Zika) could better coordinate and layer their expertise in the communities they serve. For instance, when officials learn that a disease like Zika can be sexually transmitted, they might refer to the communication and engagement centered conceptual framework to consider cultural norms around sexual intercourse, imagining how sex intersects with human rights around gender-based violence, rape, and teenage pregnancy, investigating rumors about sexual transmission of disease (including a long history of discriminatory rumors about sexual deviance in the LGBTQ community), improving ways of establishing trust between providers counseling patients about sexual and reproductive health, and confronting the complex paradigm shift of managing a vector-borne illness that can be transmitted through sex. By keeping this framework in mind as new scientific information emerges during a health emergency, responders might be better equipped to engage their communities authentically and successfully.

References

Angel-Cabo, N. (2015). Human rights legal clinics in Latin America: Tackling the implementation of disability rights. In *Disability, rights monitoring, and social change: Building power out of evidence* (pp. 97–112). Canadian Scholars' Press.

Bertrand, J. T., Ward, V. M., & Santiso Galvez Santiso, G. (2015). *Family planning in Latin America and the Caribbean: The achievements of 50 years*. MEASURE Evaluation, Carolina Population Center.

Bhatnagar, J., Rabeneck, D. B., Martines, R. B., Reagan-Steiner, S., Ermias, Y., Estetter, L. B., et al. (2017). Zika virus RNA replication and persistence in brain and placental tissue. *Emerging Infectious Diseases, 23*(3), 405.

Burger-Calderon, R., Carrillo, F. B., Gresh, L., Ojeda, S., Sanchez, N., Plazaola, M., et al. (2020). Age-dependent manifestations and case definitions of paediatric Zika: A prospective cohort study. *The Lancet Infectious Diseases, 20*(3), 371–380.

Burke, T., Kuczynski, L., & Perren, S. (2017). An exploration of Jamaican Mothers' perceptions of closeness and intimacy in the mother–child relationship during middle childhood. *Frontiers in Psychology, 8*, 2148.

CDC. (2007). *News byte. CDC global health E-brief.* Author.

Cugola, F. R., Fernandes, I. R., Russo, F. B., Freitas, B. C., Dias, J. L., Guimarães, K. P., et al. (2016). The Brazilian Zika virus strain causes birth defects in experimental models. *Nature, 534*(7606), 267–271.

Dick, G. (1952). Zika virus (II). Pathogenicity and physical properties. *Transactions of the Royal Society of Tropical Medicine, 46*(5), 521–534.

Dick, G. W., Kitchen, S., & Haddow, A. (1952). Zika virus (I). Isolations and serological specificity. *Transactions of the Royal Society of Tropical Medicine and Hygiene, 46*(5), 509–520. https://doi.org/10.1016/0035-9203(52)90042-4

Dick, O. B., San Martín, J. L., Montoya, R. H., del Diego, J., Zambrano, B., & Dayan, G. H. (2012). The history of dengue outbreaks in the Americas. *The American Journal of Tropical Medicine and Hygiene, 87*(4), 584–593.

Duffy, M. R., Chen, T. H., Hancock, W. T., Powers, A. M., Kool, J. L., Lanciotti, R. S., et al. (2009). Zika virus outbreak on Yap Island, federated states of Micronesia. *New England Journal of Medicine, 360*(24), 2536–2543.

Fagan, T., Dutta, A., Rosen, J., Olivetti, A., & Klein, K. (2017). Family planning in the context of Latin America's universal health coverage agenda. *Global Health: Science and Practice, 5*(3), 382–398.

FSM Information Services. (2007, June 26). *While HESA confirms Zika virus says quarantine unnecessary for Yap. Government of the Federated States of Micronesia Press Release*. Author.

Indar, L. (2016). *Zika and tourism*. Caribbean Public Health Organization. Retrieved from https://carpha.org/Portals/0/Documents/Zika%20Virus_Tourism.pdf

International Federation of Red Cross and Red Crescent Societies. (2017). *Knowledge, attitudes and practices around Zika in the Caribbean*. Author. Retrieved from https://www.zikacommunicationnetwork.org/

Joshi, M. P., Hafner, T., Twesigye, G., Ndiaye, A., Kiggundu, R., Mekonnen, N., et al. (2021). Strengthening multisectoral coordination on antimicrobial resistance: A landscape analysis of efforts in 11 countries. *Journal of Pharmaceutical Policy and Practice, 14*(1), 1–17.

Kieny, M. P., Rottingen, J. A., & Farrar, J. (2016). The need for global R&D coordination for infectious diseases with epidemic potential. *The Lancet, 388*(10043), 460–461.

Kindhauser, M., Allen, T., Frank, V., & Santhana, R. (2016). Zika: The origin and spread of a mosquito-borne virus. *Bulletin of the World Health Organization, 94*(9), 675–686.

Lanciotti, R. S., Kosoy, O. L., Laven, J. J., Velez, J. O., Lambert, A. J., Johnson, A. J., et al. (2008). Genetic and serologic properties of Zika virus associated with an epidemic, Yap State, Micronesia, 2007. *Emerging Infectious Diseases, 14*(8), 1232.

de Leon, R. G. P., Ewerling, F., Serruya, S. J., Silveira, M. F., Sanhueza, A., Moazzam, A., et al. (2019). Contraceptive use in Latin America and the Caribbean with a focus on long-acting reversible contraceptives: Prevalence and inequalities in 23 countries. *The Lancet Global Health, 7*(2), e227–e235.

Pan American Health Organization. (2020). *Cases of dengue in the Americas exceeded 3 million in 2019*. Author. Retrieved from https://www.paho.org/hq/index.php?option=com_content

Posada, M., Law, E., & Martes, P. (2018). *Emerging epidemics and risk perception: New evidence from Latin America and the Caribbean*. International Federation of Red Cross and Red Crescent

Societies and Save the Children. Retrieved from https://zikacommunicationnetwork.org/resources/emerging-epidemics-and-risk-perception-new-evidence-latin-america-and-caribbean

Qureshi, A. I. (2017). Economic impact of Zika virus. In *Zika virus disease: From origin to outbreak*. Academic Press. https://doi.org/10.1016/B978-0-12-812365-2.00012-3

Rossi, S. L., Ebel, G. D., Shan, C., Shi, P. Y., & Vasilakis, N. (2018). Did Zika virus mutate to cause severe outbreaks? *Trends in Microbiology, 26*(10), 877–885.

Samms-Vaughan, M. E., Williams, S., & Brown, J. (2005). Disciplinary practices among parents of six year olds in Jamaica. *Caribbean Childhoods: From Research to Action, 2*, 58–70.

Satterfield-Nash, A., Kotzky, K., Allen, J., Bertolli, J., Moore, C. A., Pereira, I. O., et al. (2017). Health and development at age 19–24 months of 19 children who were born with microcephaly and laboratory evidence of congenital Zika virus infection during the 2015 Zika virus outbreak—Brazil, 2017. *MMWR. Morbidity and Mortality Weekly Report, 66*(49), 1347.

Smith, D. E., & Moore, T. M. (2013). Parenting style and psychosocial outcomes in a sample of Jamaican adolescents. *International Journal of Adolescence and Youth, 18*(3), 176–190.

Smith, D. E., & Mosby, G. (2003). Jamaican child-rearing practices: The role of corporal punishment. *Adolescence, 38*(150), 369.

Smithburn, K. (1952). Neutralizing antibodies against certain recently isolated viruses in the sera of human beings residing in East Africa. *The Journal of Immunology, 69*(2), 223–234.

Southwell, B. G., Dolina, S., Jimenez-Magdaleno, K., Squiers, L. B., & Kelly, B. J. (2016). Zika virus-related news coverage and online behavior, United States, Guatemala, and Brazil. *Emerging Infectious Diseases, 22*(7), 1320–1321. https://doi.org/10.3201/eid2207.160415

Steely, A. C., & Rohner, R. P. (2006). Relations among corporal punishment, perceived parental acceptance, and psychological adjustment in Jamaican youths. *Cross-Cultural Research, 40*(3), 268–286.

United Nations Development Programme. (2017). *A socio-economic impact assessment of the Zika virus in Latin America and the Caribbean: With a focus on Brazil, Colombia and Suriname*. Author.

URC. (2020). *USAID Applying Science to Strengthen and Improve Systems (ASSIST) project – Country summaries*. Author. Retrieved from https://www.urc-chs.com/sites/default/files/USAID%20ASSIST%20Project%20-%20Country%20Summaries.pdf

Van der Linden, V., Pessoa, A., Dobyns, W., Barkovich, A. J., van der Linden Júnior, H., Filho, E. L. R., et al. (2016). Description of 13 infants born during October 2015–January 2016 with congenital Zika virus infection without microcephaly at birth—Brazil. *Morbidity and Mortality Weekly Report, 65*(47), 1343–1348.

World Health Organization. (2016). *Knowledge, attitudes and practice surveys Zika virus disease and potential complications. Emergency preparedness, response*. Author. Retrieved from https://www.who.int/csr/resources/publications/zika/kap-surveys/en/

Yactayo, S., Staples, J. E., Millot, V., Cibrelus, L., & Ramon-Pardo, P. (2016). Epidemiology of Chikungunya in the Americas. *The Journal of Infectious Diseases, 214*(suppl_5), S441–S445.

Yuan, L., Huang, X. Y., Liu, Z. Y., Zhang, F., Zhu, X. L., Yu, J. Y., et al. (2017). A single mutation in the prM protein of Zika virus contributes to fetal microcephaly. *Science, 358*(6365), 933–936.

Chapter 8
An Experiential Account of the Risk Communication and Community Engagement Early Response to the COVID-19 Pandemic in Chile and Paraguay: Lessons and Recommendations

Paolo Mefalopulos and Rafael Obregon

Contents

Introduction

By early August 2020, almost 18 million confirmed cases of Coronavirus-19 (COVID-19) and over 670,000 deaths had been reported worldwide across more than 210 countries and territories. The USA remained the country with the most cases (4.6 million) followed by Brazil (2.6 million) (Johns Hopkins University, 2021). Latin America had become the epicenter of the pandemic with Mexico, Peru, Chile, Colombia, and Argentina also reporting significant numbers of confirmed cases and implementing prolonged quarantine measures. Latin America also

P. Mefalopulos
UNICEF, Santiago, Chile

R. Obregon (✉)
UNICEF, Asunción, Paraguay
e-mail: robregon@unicef.org

E. Manoncourt et al. (eds.), *Communication and Community Engagement in Disease Outbreaks*, https://doi.org/10.1007/978-3-030-92296-2_8

included countries with relatively contained COVID-19 outbreaks, especially Uruguay, Nicaragua, Cuba, and Paraguay.

In this chapter, we provide an experiential account and analysis of the communication and community engagement dimensions of the Chile and Paraguay responses to the COVID-19 pandemic, with a particular focus on the first few months of the emergency. The COVID-19 pandemic has challenged science and key concepts such as evidence-based interventions, but it also provides opportunities to learn and improve preparedness and response in the long run. The respective experiences of Chile and Paraguay provide relevant and complementary insights and lessons that can inform future responses. Their responses were permeated, and often defined, by multiple factors beyond the public health domain, in line with the conceptual framework discussed in Chap. 1. Our analysis is by no means exhaustive; however, as we recognize the great levels of uncertainty and the rapidly changing science and evidence of COVID-19, we do believe that our account contributes to the massive literature about the role of communication and community engagement in this pandemic and beyond.

Experiential accounts and analysis are commonly used in qualitative research. They focus on the interaction and immersion of researchers in a specific reality which leads to an ongoing series of reflections about that reality, informed by the researchers' current and past experiences (Reinharz, 1983). While this is not a research undertaking in the strict sense, for our analysis we examine: (a) the intersection of social, political, and economic factors of the response and its communicative dimensions; and (b) the relevance of public and community trust as a core dimension of the COVID-19 response. We, specifically, draw upon: (a) our direct engagement in the COVID-19 response in Chile and Paraguay, respectively; and (b) our previous and extensive experience in supporting the communication and community engagement dimension of several responses to public health emergencies of international concern (Public Health Emergencies of International Concern - PHEIC -, i.e., H1N1, Ebola Virus Disease, Zika Virus) and to pandemic and disease outbreak preparedness and response (i.e., Human Immunodeficiency Virus - HIV-, polio, dengue) in several regions of the world.

Chile, with a population of 17.5 million, is a high-income country and one of Latin America's fastest-growing economies in recent decades which has enabled poverty reduction. Between 2000 and 2015, the population living in poverty decreased from 20.2% to 8.6%. However, inequity, reflected throughout all sectors of society, remains Chile's major challenge. In October 2019, Chile was rocked by social unrest and mass demonstrations, damage to property, and looting triggered by Chile's severe inequalities. This led to the Government's decision, supported by most political parties, to hold a referendum for a new constitution, as demanded by protesters. Chile's first confirmed case of COVID-19 was reported on March 3, 2020 and on March 15, the country experienced a sharp rise in cases from 14 to 81[1] in just 1 day. On March 18, Chile's president, Sebastian Piñera, declared "the state

[1] Gobierno de Chile (n.d.). Cifras Oficiales Covid-19. Gob.cl - Cifras Oficiales (www.gob.cl).

of catastrophe" for 90 days, an extraordinary measure subsequently extended for another 90 days. By June 2020, Chile ranked third in COVID-19 cases in Latin America.

While Paraguay also experienced steady economic growth over the past two decades and reduced poverty from 41% to 28% by 2013, still about 1.8 million people, out of a total population of 7.1 million, live in poverty. Also, more than 50% of the workforce of the country works in the informal sector, which makes them highly vulnerable to any negative changes in the economy or to the emergence of political or health crises. In August 2019, just a few months before the pandemic, the country faced a political crisis and a stagnant economy, along with one of the worst dengue outbreaks in recent history, which eventually, as discussed later in this chapter, influenced key decisions in the response to COVID-19.

Paraguay reported its first confirmed case of COVID-19 on March 10, 2020. Immediately after, the government announced a nationwide quarantine and strict physical isolation measures, including the closing of schools, one of the first countries in the region to take such measures. The introduction of these measures so early in the response were primarily driven by the need to strengthen the limited capacity of the country's health systems, already overwhelmed by one of the most severe dengue outbreaks in many years. Other measures introduced over time included the closing of the country's borders with Brazil and Argentina, areas of great mobility and commercial activity, the suspension of commercial flights in and out of the country, and the setup of albergues (provisional quarantine centers) in the border areas to cope with the return of the increasing number of Paraguayans living in Brazil and Argentina.

In the following sections of this chapter, we provide a brief overview of the early response of both countries to the pandemic; discuss the social, economic, and political context in each country and how it informed communication and community engagement dimensions of their responses; examine the critical role of trust in the response; and put forward several recommendations for ongoing and future responses.

Early Country Responses: The Local and the National

Despite similarities in terms of how Chile and Paraguay entered the COVID-19 pandemic, their responses in the first few months differed considerably and led to different outcomes. The social, economic, and political context in which COVID-19 surfaced in both the countries was already very complex due to the social unrest and political crises they experienced at different times before and throughout the emergency. What began as a protest against the hike in the metro fare in Santiago de Chile, for instance, soon spread throughout the country and turned into riots, looting and incidents that resulted in several metro stations badly damaged, supermarkets set on fire, and the deaths of at least 24 people in the first few weeks of protests. The metro fare hike was simply the detonator of the wider social discontent that, at its core, included the high cost of living and the severe socio-economic inequalities of the Chilean society (BBC News, 2020). While this type of demonstrations was not part of Paraguay's experience in the first few months of the response, social discontent was already present since August 2019, when the current government faced a political crisis that jeopardized its continuity. After a few months of success in the early part of the response in 2020, social discontent continued to rise and it gradually led to mass demonstrations and to demands for changes in the government (Carneri & Politi, 2021), which eventually led to the replacement of the ministers of health and education.

Following the initial country lockdown, the Chilean government adopted a selected containment or "dynamic quarantine" strategy, a decision driven by the perceived risks (financial and social) of prolonging the lockdown for too long and by the potential negative implications on people's mental health. A dynamic quarantine meant that, based upon epidemiological data, municipalities[2] with a higher infection rate had to implement measures such as sanitary confinement, use of masks, and online permits to allow citizens to leave their homes. Criteria to decide whether to place a municipality in quarantine included the number of cases in the previous 2 weeks, the fragility of its health system, and the social vulnerability of the residents (Martínez et al., 2020). Municipalities that showed sustained improvement in the epidemiological curve could exit from the quarantine while others with a rising curve would enter it.

Several social actors questioned the dynamic "quarantine" due to challenges in traceability and mobility containment (Miranda, 2020). Municipalities adjacent to each other, for instance, could have different epidemiological profiles that made it virtually impossible to monitor people's movements. Some municipalities initially put in quarantine, exited it after a couple of weeks, only to reenter soon after, which created a sense of disorientation among the public. The dynamic quarantine made difficult the implementation of a comprehensive communication strategy at national and local levels, as municipalities, even within the same urban area, adopted different measures during the same period. Chile's declaration of the state of emergency also meant a national curfew from 22.00 to 05.00 h, the closure of schools, and the postponement of the constitutional referendum originally set to October 25, 2020. Those measures, however, were not always followed by clear messaging by public health authorities. The easing of the restrictive measures in April, such as the gradual opening of seven municipalities and the "Safe Return Plan," for instance, implied the return of students and workers and the re-opening of commercial activities. This resulted in tensions with local mayors and the subsequent increase in daily cases led again to the application of more restrictive measures.

According to some critics, the limited success in containing the early rise in infections should be mostly ascribed to the ambivalent messaging by the Ministry

[2] Chile territory is subdivided in "comunas," which are administrative units that can be roughly compared to municipalities, each with its own elected mayor. For instance, Santiago, the capital of the country, is composed by 32 comunas or municipalities, while Greater Santiago, that is the whole metropolitan region, has 52.

of Health, which ranged from a strong confidence in the capacity to control the epidemic, mostly in March and April 2020, to a manifest pessimism as the number of cases increased, often blamed on the public's lack of adherence to the recommended behaviors (Araya, 2020). Between March and May 2020, several measures were implemented across the country and communicated to audiences via mass media and social media. However, analysts pointed to the limited consistency in messaging and the challenges of the "dynamic quarantine approach" as factors that did not contribute to communicating effectively with the public (Araya, 2020; Martínez et al., 2020). Depending upon the epidemiological status of the municipalities, recommendations were understood very differently, a likely cause for the limited acceptance and adoption of preventative behaviors.

Although by August 2020 Chile was performing the highest number of Polymerase Chain Reaction (PCR) tests in the region and had added extra capacity to its health system, the increase in the number of COVID-19 cases in that period highlighted not only the challenges of the government's response but also the limitations in implementing an effective communication strategy to promote rapid behavior changes. The decision to adopt a dynamic quarantine in Chile, as opposed to a total lockdown, as it was done in many countries including Paraguay, hindered the implementation of a homogeneous communication campaign across the country. Different municipalities implemented different measures that, in turn, required adherence to different behaviors, including washing hands, covering mouth and nose, and maintaining physical distancing, but the fact that they were mandatory in some places while only recommended in others did not help to establish these behaviors as the norm.

Paraguay's response plan to COVID-19 followed the WHO guidelines which outline the key response pillars (World Health Organization, 2020), including the activation of the Emergency Operations Center (EOC) (World Health Organization, 2020). Immediately after the confirmation of the first COVID-19 case in the country, the government introduced restrictive measures such as a nationwide lockdown for 14 days, extended several times over a 3-month period, and put in place standard disease outbreak guidelines—early detection of suspected cases, contact tracing and isolation, and care for the ill. Because of these measures, along with others such as the closing of borders with Brazil and Argentina, and the suspension of commercial flights and of all public activities, the circulation of the COVID-19 virus was very limited throughout the first 6 months of the pandemic. As stated above, the implementation of these measures so early was driven primarily by the need to buy time to strengthen the country's health system capacity, including for laboratory testing, construction of new hospitals and more hospital beds, more ICUs, and training of healthcare personnel, among others.

The Ministry of Health and Social Welfare activated the Risk Communication and Community Engagement (RCCE) pillar, in charge of communicating with the public about risk behaviors and preventive practices, promoting early care-seeking behaviors, and building public trust in the response. During the first 6 months, this pillar primarily focused on the dissemination of critical information about control and prevention measures including social distancing, handwashing, reporting of symptoms to the emergency toll-free number, physical isolation at home, timely care-seeking in case of worsening conditions, and, eventually, the use of masks in public places. Some of the most effective communication actions included the Minister of Health's daily updates, through his Twitter account, that listed the number of new cases, the number of patients hospitalized, and the number of deaths due to COVID-19. The Minister's Twitter followers increased from only a few thousand in January 2020 to nearly half a million by July 2020 (La Nación, 2020).

The Minister's weekly press briefings were broadcast by all TV channels and radio stations in the country, which contributed early on to building public trust in the government's response. A survey on public perceptions conducted by UNICEF in mid-May 2020 showed that 90% of respondents viewed the Ministry of Health as the most trusted source of information about COVID-19, and the majority of respondents indicated that they were satisfied with the information provided by the government thus far (see Fig. 8.1).

Although Paraguay performed a very limited number of PCR tests throughout 2020, the fact that it consistently reported a very low number of confirmed cases throughout the first few months of the pandemic was seen both by the public and by the global health community as an example of an effective and successful response (Goni & Costa, 2020).

The experiences of Chile and Paraguay in the first few months of the response provide an interesting contrast of local and national approaches and RCCE strategies that led to different epidemiological outcomes. The differentiating factor in both cases was, to a large extent, the social, political, and economic context in which the response took place, which in turn had a significant impact on how communities

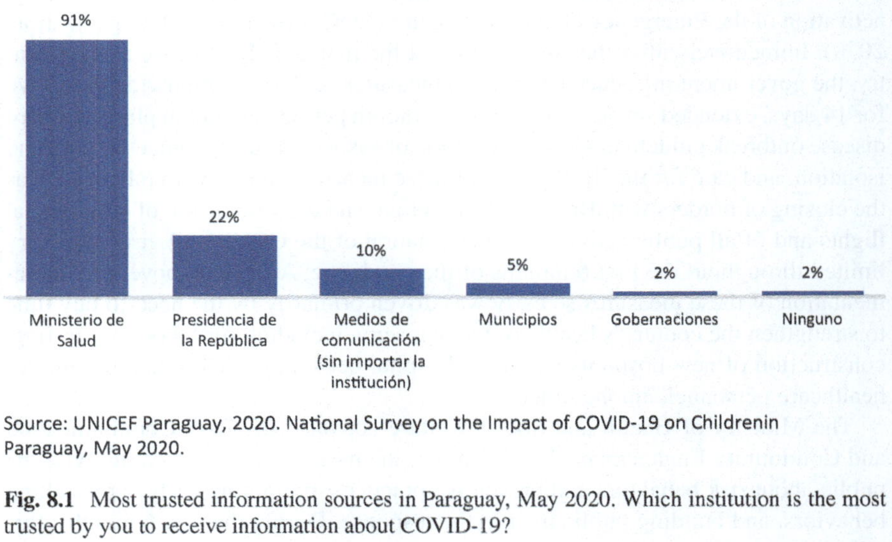

Fig. 8.1 Most trusted information sources in Paraguay, May 2020. Which institution is the most trusted by you to receive information about COVID-19?

perceived the risks associated with the virus, adopted (or did not adopt) key behaviors, and engaged with the government and public health authorities, especially in terms of their trust in the response.

Social, Economic, and Political Context

The socio-economic and political realities of Chile and Paraguay intersected regularly, clearly, and directly with key aspects of the communication and engagement component of the response. We discuss these issues in more depth in this section. We have clustered the social, economic, and political issues that influenced communication and community engagement in Chile and Paraguay into three domains—public policy, organizational, and socio-cultural.

The public policy dimension refers to decisions taken by the governments to address the COVID-19 emergency and the related budget allocated to implement those policies. Implementation of the state of emergency, the application of unemployment insurance, the allocation of bonuses and family emergency income, the expansion of cash transfer programs, among others, are policy-related measures that sought to mitigate the impact of the pandemic on the lower socio-economic sectors of society (Valcarcel et al., 2020). The Government of Chile enacted such measures to alleviate the economic difficulties experienced by the most vulnerable groups. These measures included unemployment insurance, a COVID-19 bonus that reached 2.7 million vulnerable people, family emergency income, food baskets, and other basic goods for vulnerable families. However, they were not enough to cover everyone. The socio-economic consequences of the pandemic quickly became very severe and the initial estimates of recession, the fall of the gross domestic product (GDP), and the rise of unemployment exceeded all previous projections.

While the number of confirmed COVID-19 cases in Paraguay remained very low throughout the first few months of the pandemic, compared to the rest of the region, the measures introduced to contain the spread of the virus quickly impacted many people, especially the most vulnerable. The government provided economic relief to nearly 400,000 families through a cash transfer program, the delivery of lunches to school children and to families enrolled in social protection programs, loans to small- and medium-sized businesses, and the suspension of collection of fees for energy services for at least 3 months, among others. Most of these programs, however, were short-lived due to the urgent need for substantive investments in strengthening the country's public health system. In that context, it quickly became very difficult for most informal workers and small businesses in Paraguay to remain in isolation or closed without a reliable source of income, which in turn impacted upon people's ability to comply with key behaviors such as physical and social distancing, regular handwashing, and mask wearing.

The measures implemented by the governments of Chile and Paraguay underscored the sense of emergency due to COVID-19, but they also highlighted the difficulties that poorer people, whose livelihoods were at risk, faced in order to comply with the recommended behaviors.

The organizational dimension focuses on how state institutions, civil society organizations, community-led organizations, foundations, academic centers, and private sector groups reacted to the emergency. Health institutions, public and private, begun preparing even before the virus was first announced in Chile. Health workers, who have worked hard throughout the pandemic, at times expressed some frustration about how the messaging was handled in the early phase of the response. The main health workers' union, for instance, had tense relations with the Minister of Health, Jaime Mañalich, partially due to some of his controversial statements (Miranda, 2020), which were perceived to make a coherent approach to messaging over the severity of the virus very challenging. Those factors, combined with the difficulty to control mobility and to monitor traceability of cases, eventually contributed to the resignation of the minister by mid-June 2020. In parallel, many civil society organizations increased their activities to support the most vulnerable, and the private sector undertook different initiatives to soften the impact of the pandemic. While COVID-19 negatively affected the social and economic environment of society, it also strengthened the sense of solidarity in the community.

Following the declaration of the state of emergency, the Chilean government ordered a national curfew and sent the army into the streets, a decision that concerned many citizens due to the country's recent history of military dictatorship. While this and other measures taken to restrict mass gatherings reduced the number and the intensity of the protests, many felt that the Government saw it as an opportunity to address and contain the possible revamp of widespread protests. On October 25, 2020, over a million people participated in a mass demonstration that was labeled as the biggest of modern times in Chile. As stated earlier, such mass gatherings often created an enabling environment for the rapid spread of the virus.

Paraguay imposed strict measures from Day 1 of the response and in parallel launched national communication campaigns to explain how the virus was spreading and what behaviors were key to minimize the risk of contagion, including the message "quedate en casa" (stay at home), which had both intended and unintended consequences. The messaging of these campaigns was further enforced by the authorities as they initially sanctioned those who did not comply with the recommended behaviors (i.e., breaking the curfew). This strict approach was meant not only to delay the spread of the contagion but also to buy time to strengthen the health system to eventually cope with a spike in cases. Paraguay was largely successful with this approach up until early September 2020. By then, it had recorded only about 412 deaths due to the COVID-19.

Throughout the first few months of the pandemic, numerous civil society organizations engaged in extraordinary efforts to support vulnerable families, especially through the distribution of basic supplies (i.e., soap, masks, alcohol) and the implementation of the *ollas populares* (community kitchens) that typically help feed 50 or so families per community. And while the ollas populares, which during a brief period of time received financial subsidies from the government, helped thousands of families to access at least one meal a day, they also have several limitations in terms of their long-term sustainability, the nutritional value of the meals, and the increase in the risk of exposure to the virus and potential contagion for the community leaders and members.

The third dimension refers to the **social context**, including the norms, cultural habits, and behaviors that can facilitate or impede the spread of the virus. Social discontent is usually expressed through mass protests that draw people to march in the streets, likely in close physical proximity of each other. Even if protests in Chile were greatly reduced over time, they likely contributed to the spread of the virus. Similarly, social gatherings in which there was little or no concern for physical distancing and for mask-wearing became increasingly frequent, especially among youth, even in municipalities in a state of lockdown. Police often intervened and closed several private parties that ignored the preventative measures, especially in the metropolitan region. In Paraguay, the sustainability of physical and social distancing and mask-wearing became very challenging, but for different reasons. Despite warnings about the need to not let their guard down, for instance, the low number of cases and deaths throughout the first few months of the pandemic conveyed a false sense of security and lower levels of perceived risks, especially among younger people.

The increase in COVID-19 cases throughout the first several months of 2020 in Chile highlighted the challenges of the response, and particularly of the implementation of an effective communication strategy to promote changes in behaviors needed to mitigate the risk of contagion. Among the many social norms and behaviors that needed to be changed was the way to greet each other. In Chile, as in most Latin-American countries, it is normal to greet family and friends by hugging and kissing each other on the cheek. However, kissing and hugging were frequently observable for several weeks after the pandemic had started and even during the period when the number of cases began to rise. In Paraguay, the consumption of "terere," a practice heavily ingrained in the Paraguayan culture and through which two or more people, often family members or groups of friends, drink from the same pot a cold infusion made of local herbs, raised concerns as it lends itself to widespread transmission of viruses. Sharing of terere means trust, community-building, friendship, and bonding, while rejecting terere is often frowned upon and may even be considered an offense among certain groups (Boswell, 2017). "Preparing tereré ... is a communal tradition. Families drink it together on weekend outings. Ministry officials share it while planning meetings. The bus driver passes it to the restless passenger behind him" (Boswell, 2017).

From the start of the pandemic, consumption of terere was identified as a key source of transmission. Messages about the risks associated with this practice were emphasized in communication campaigns. Yet, all throughout the response, it has been clear that individuals and community groups continue to engage in this practice. Countless pictures and videos have circulated through broadcast media and other social media platforms that show people of all ages and socio-economic backgrounds sharing terere. Because the number of COVID-19 cases in Paraguay remained low through the first few months of the pandemic, the practice of terere did not seem to have a significant impact on transmission of the virus. However, as the number of cases rose in July 2020 (to nearly 20,000), terere regained considerable attention (Ministerio de Salud y Bienestar Social de Paraguay, 2020).

In summary, the social, economic, and political context in both the countries played, and continues to play, a very important role in the promotion of key behaviors to prevent and control the spread of COVID-19. In addition to the challenges posed by the normalized behaviors (i.e., greetings with hugs and kisses, consumption of terere), adherence to social distancing was a major challenge, particularly in Chile, due to the mass protests and the rooted cultural habits such as close physical proximity and contact in social interactions. Similarly, over time, in both Chile and Paraguay, economic constrains made it very difficult to comply with the recommended behaviors, especially the messages "stay at home" or those focused on maintaining physical distancing, as considerable numbers of people, especially in the lower socio-economic strata, had to leave their homes to make a daily living. In Paraguay, data from the UNICEF survey on the impact of COVID-19 showed that 57% of respondents indicated that the primary reason to leave their homes was "going to work."

While recognizing the role of the socio-political and economic context of Chile and Paraguay as key to the successful implementation of RCCE strategies should not come as a surprise, it is less clear the extent to which those strategies took social and contextual factors into account and how they influenced, or not, the adoption of the preventative behaviors. Further, as in the case of Paraguay, messages such as "stay at home" had unintended consequences, particularly with regard to care-seeking behaviors for other equally important health issues such as immunization and maternal and child health services. As it has been the case in other pandemics or in large outbreaks, a focus on key messages driven primarily by biomedical considerations often misses critical social, political, and economic issues that play a much bigger role in people's decisions and in shaping RCCE strategies.

Public and Community Trust: Building and Sustaining It

Adherence to recommended behaviors in public health, especially in the context of disease outbreaks and pandemics of rapid onset, is highly interconnected with the level of trust that the public, communities, and individuals have in the government and in social service providers (Siegrist & Zingg, 2014). And the reputation and credibility of the messenger is an important factor for the public and communities to adhere to recommended behaviors, especially if these are new. The COVID-19 experience of Chile and Paraguay reiterate the important role of trust in disease outbreak and pandemic response. Mody (1991) put forward six key elements for defining messages for behavior change: sociocultural sensitivity, language appropriateness, political compatibility, economic compatibility, psychological appropriateness, and expected achievements. Chile's experience highlighted another key element, namely the need for message cohesiveness and coherence which eventually hurt public trust.

In Chile, three interconnected issues impacted trust-building in the first few months of the response. First, the conflicting messages from state authorities. Public commitment is a means to build trust (Bicchieri, 2017), and trust requires a consistent process with consistent messages. The conflicting messages disseminated by the health authorities in Chile, for instance, often alerted the population about the gravity of the situation but at times they also conveyed an optimistic overtone, which may have weakened the effectiveness of the messages about the preventative behaviors. Second, the difficulty of applying a RCCE strategy flexible enough to support the territorial diversification needed for the dynamic quarantine approach also affected message effectiveness. Changes in key messages from scientific sources and the proliferation of fake news and conspiracy theories that circulate on the web have damaged the public's trust in science and have made effective communication of factual knowledge more challenging. Third, despite the wide availability of mass media and social media, the segmentation of audiences based on restricted geographical boundaries also proved to be a major constraint that could not be easily overcome.

The Paraguay response to the COVID-19 pandemic had an interesting trajectory throughout the first few months. In the early phase of the response, the Minister of Health and, broadly speaking, the "trabajadores de blanco" (health workers) became akin to national heroes for keeping the spread of the virus under control. Through the first 2 months of the pandemic, largely due to the valiant measures taken by the government such as the national lockdown and closure of borders and school, the number of cases remained as one of the lowest worldwide, leading to international praise (The Guardian, 2020; Treader, 2020). The Ministry of Health (MOH) emphasized to the public that strict measures were needed not only to protect themselves and their own families and communities but also to buy time to strengthen the capacity of the healthcare system and mount a more effective response. The UNICEF survey on citizens' perceptions about the impact of the response conducted in May 2020 showed that the Minister of Health was the most trusted source of health information (92%).

As the pandemic progressed, however, the limited capacity of the Paraguay's MOH to handle procurement demands and other logistical aspects of the response began to weaken public trust. Media reports denounced that some suppliers of medical equipment had not complied with government requirements and that they had insiders' connections to access contracts. This led to a public outcry that started to question the credibility of the MOH and their teams (The Guardian, 2020). While most analyses pointed out that it was important to make a distinction between the technical role of the MOH and whether it had effectively handled the response and the managerial aspects of it, it was difficult to detach the technical role from the responsibilities of managing huge amounts of resources, to the tune of more than US$500 million from a World Bank loan that were not spent in a timely manner or were seen as subject to corrupt practices that have plagued the country's public system for years (Carnieri and Politi, 2021).

While it is key to enter a pandemic or outbreak with considerable public trust, it is even more critical to maintain it throughout, especially in a prolonged response such as in the case of COVID-19. In Paraguay, the situation described earlier and several others (for instance, perceptions that special treatment was being given to powerful political figures) gradually eroded public trust in the government and health authorities. (Carnieri and Polit, 2021)This was capped by the resignation of one of the MOH's vice ministers due to his participation in a party that violated quarantine restrictions, of which pictures and a brief video went viral on social media. While the primary focus of trust-building in the early phase of the response emphasized biomedical issues and government efforts to address the socio-economic needs of the more vulnerable populations, it did not take too long for the socio-economic impact of the response measures and the public perceptions of administrative mismanagement to show in the social fabric of the country.

As small businesses started to shut down, people started to lose jobs while informal workers, who make up more than 50% of the workforce in Paraguay, increasingly had to leave their homes to work and to make ends meet. In essence, the strict quarantine and social isolation measures were harder to maintain. The government ran into difficulties in maintaining social protection programs for a long period of time, while community members, business networks, and informal workers began to defy compliance with public health measures (ADN Digital, 2020). The role of these socio-economic dynamics of the response reveals that trust-building in pandemic response is not fully dependent upon the response of the health sector only. Instead, it clearly needs to consider a wide range of issues early on, which should be fully integrated into pandemic preparedness and response plans. What are the socio-economic implications of disease outbreaks? What issues need to be assessed and eventually addressed in order to minimize their impact? How could these issues impact trust?

As stated previously, in the early phase of the response, the RCCE pillar in Paraguay primarily focused on identifying key messages and communicating those through official channels. In practical terms, the RCCE pillar was not fully operational and the lack of a strong focus on community engagement was increasingly felt. While the initial focus on communicating risk worked well, over time fatigue started to set in, and people´s trust started to weaken and to engage in behaviors that increased their risk of infection. The UNICEF survey on perceptions about the impact of the pandemic in Paraguay showed that more than 50% of the population between 18 and 45 years of age believed that it was very unlikely that they or someone in their family would contract COVID-19, which meant that perceived susceptibility was considerably low. By October 2020, the number of daily confirmed cases in the country skyrocketed to nearly 1000 per day, with a considerably higher case fatality rate of people hospitalized due to COVID-19 complications.

Building and sustaining trust in the first few months of the Chile and Paraguay responses to the COVID-19 pandemic is an interesting case of somewhat contrasting scenarios. Despite the strict measures that Paraguay introduced, the Ministry of Health was able to build strong public trust and support, while Chile had the opposite experience. However, over time, public trust in Paraguay declined while Chile was able to build it back up again. These dynamics not only reveal important lessons about trust-building and the need to sustain it over time but also about how social, political, economic, cultural, behavioral, and communicative issues intersect and determine key outcomes of the response.

Implications and Recommendations for Future Preparedness/ Response

The experience of Chile and Paraguay highlights several important lessons and issues. In dealing with a pandemic of this nature, a linear communication approach is not very effective. Instead, such challenge calls for a multidimensional, multi-audience, and multimedia approach. Multidimensional means that actions need to be considered and applied in each of the three dimensions discussed earlier—policy, organizational, and social context, including a focus on norms and culture. RCCE strategies should take into consideration policy measures, allocation of budgets, preparation and strengthening of health institutions, alliances of different organizations to support social and economic measures for vulnerable households, and campaigns and communication initiatives to influence positive changes in cultural norms and individual behaviors (Gerber et al., 2021).

Multi-audience refers to the need of carefully segmenting audiences and investigating the needs, perceptions, drivers, and appeals of each one of them, an aspect that many agencies and governments are increasingly paying attention to through initiatives focused on strengthening the contribution of social and behavioral sciences, including approaches such as behavioral insights. We know, for instance, that youth often engage in high-risk behaviors because their perception of risk and of perceived vulnerability may be quite different compared to older people. That was one of the reasons why anti-smoking campaigns that had success with the overall population tended to fail when applied to teens and younger audiences.

In the case of COVID-19, evidence shows that perceived risk among young people has remained considerably low. It is critical to take these factors into account when designing RCCE strategies and messages. For instance, it is worth asking who has more persuasive influence on youth, whether a renowned epidemiologist or a peer? Tina Rosenberg in her book *Join the Club: How Peer Pressure Can Transform the World* (Rosenberg, 2011) presents several examples and compelling evidence on how peer pressure in young audiences is the most effective way, if not the only one, to promote adoption of new behaviors. However, peer influence has not been adopted to any significant scale in persuading young people to comply with the recommended behaviors against COVID-19. It seems that among youth, the tipping point (Gladwell, 2000) has not been reached, thus making it difficult to switch to the recommended behaviors.

Finally, the multi-media approach refers to the mix of mass media and community engagement activities such as broadcast and social media, which have been segmented, profiled, and probed in advance, as well as the type of community-level interactions that lend themselves to dialogue and trust. Social media, however, present an additional challenge. While interactivity provides individuals with the possibility of being senders and recipients of information at the same time, they are also susceptible to being targeted with or exposed to false and incorrect information, a core aspect of the infodemics dimension discussed in this book. The role of fake news makes people's compliance with mitigating measures more difficult. The segmentation of and the regular engagement with audiences is a critical point in preparedness (Siegrist & Zingg, 2014). This should be accompanied by an evidence-based profiling, and the identification of the most influential sources of information for each group and of their own community-based communication spaces. In these times of media overload, the message is not necessarily more important than the messenger. The credibility and proximity of the messenger to the groups of reference can make a significant difference in their decision to adopt to or to negotiate new behaviors. This aspect may have not been adequately explored in the Chile and Paraguay experiences, and it should be considered in future emergencies (Gerber et al., 2021).

The Chile and Paraguay experiences reiterate the need to develop systems and capacities to pre-position and craft coherent strategies and messages about recommended behaviors prior to the outbreak or from the very beginning, depending on the type of disease. We have learned through the years that the adoption of any new behavior is a challenging task because it depends upon several interrelated communication factors, including the source of the messages, the context where the change is expected to occur, the channels being used and through which the messages are disseminated and the characteristics of the audience. Based on our experience, we summarize several communication factors and their implications. The Chilean experience shows that different messages addressing different localities in a rapidly changing context is a considerable challenge, and it is likely to dilute message effectiveness.

As stated earlier, audience segmentation by age is a key criterium in the COVID-19 response not only because of the greater susceptibility of older people but also because differences in risk perceptions across age may contribute to the rapid spread of the virus (e.g., young people may be more likely to congregate in closed spaces such as bars, discos). Gender is another important factor to be considered. We know that COVID-19 seems to be more aggressive with men, but also the way COVID-19 impacts families determines how they, especially women, engage in or support the adoption of preventative behaviors. Therefore, the appeals for promoting changes in behaviors need to be gender-sensitive. This observation also applies to other vulnerability factors such as disability and ethnicity. Based on our analysis, however, this type of segmentation for communication purposes has been, for the most part, absent.

Our analysis also highlights the importance of the messengers. While the national health authorities must be among the main messengers, especially with regard to critical messages about the science of the virus, they, alone, may not be enough to influence key changes in behaviors or to maintain a considerable level of influence over a long period of time in rapidly evolving pandemics such as COVID-19. Other credible messengers can enhance opportunities to engage and dialogue with different audiences about changes in or negotiation of behaviors. Diversification of voices, especially for community engagement, should be a critical consideration.

Evidence shows that a mix of channels is usually more effective than the use of a single medium. Effectiveness increases if the channel mix includes an interpersonal communication component that is dialogue-based and community-centered. Channels' features and their popularity with different audience groups need to be carefully assessed when deciding the communication strategy. While this is widely known, there remains a tendency to default to a predetermined combination of channels to prioritize wide dissemination of key messages, in place of community-based channels that can lead to greater frequency of interaction with individuals and communities.

Existing norms and behaviors are critical in facilitating or impeding the adoption of the new behaviors; therefore, an assessment of cultural norms and beliefs, habits and current behaviors must guide RCCE decisions. The example of the consumption of terere in Paraguay illustrates the potential impact it can have as a potential source of infection for the ongoing pandemic or for new ones. While messages that focus on not sharing the terere cup (guampa) have been widely disseminated, the promotion of alternative or negotiated behaviors has not been equally prevalent. Community-based solutions should be identified, ideally before a new wave of the virus hits or before a new, highly transmissible virus emerges, to ensure that drinking tereres remain at the heart of Paraguayan culture but also in a way that does not contribute to transmission of the virus.

When the measures to reduce the spread of the virus are not medical or pharmaceutical but behavioral, trust is key to ensuring that messages can have the intended persuasion effectiveness. Trust is required if audiences are expected to place confidence in the soundness of scientific data and in the spokespersons of scientific knowledge. However, different groups of people place their trust in different sources and science is not always the main driver of their decisions, as the experiences of Paraguay and Chile and the rise of fake news illustrate. In Chile and Paraguay, public health authorities have faced ups and downs regarding trust and credibility. On the other hand, fake news indicate that facts are increasingly evaluated against the value system of the audiences, thus scientific truth and factual reality often become less important than the source of the messages.

In Paraguay, the decline in trust in the authorities over time has affected the effectiveness of communication strategies, while increased community engagement through local leaders and community volunteers have become extremely valuable in supporting the promotion of critical behaviors. What this tells us is that trust is a dynamic value that needs to be continuously cultivated. Different audience groups can have different rankings about who is trustworthy and credible, a critical reason for defining and segmenting audiences before selecting the most effective messengers. As many individuals appear to be more inclined to trust and believe news according to their socio-political affinity with the source, RCCE strategies need to evolve to take these factors into account. If information and knowledge are no longer a direct reflection of truth, but of subjective interpretation or of the interpretation of a given messenger, then this requires a significant shift in the design of a communication strategy. It is no longer enough to ensure that the message is evidence-based, factually correct and has the appropriate appeal. To be effective, the message should also be disseminated by a trusted source, somebody who is credible and whose worldview can resonate with that of the intended audience. This may be hard to do in some cases, but it may be an unavoidable task.

An important source of resistance to adopting protective measures and behaviors has come from groups who have denounced some of these behaviors as limiting their individual rights, an issue that has been raised in Chap. 1 and is mentioned earlier in this chapter. This should be carefully but inevitably addressed. Is the requirement to wear a mask a violation of individual rights? Is the prohibition of mass gatherings another violation? The need to identify sources or champions with a high degree of credibility and who can talk to and reach different audiences is high, especially in pandemic contexts. For many others, restrictions need to be negotiated with the affected communities to the extent possible as they may be seen as violations of their rights. Are lockdowns and prolonged quarantines sustainable without stronger social protection programs in place? Are school closures viable without proper alternatives to continuity of education and learning, especially for children? What is the balance, if any, between individual rights and the social good? How does the world better prepare for such situations? Different groups put their trust in different sources.

In this chapter, we sought to provide an experiential account and analysis of the communication and community engagement dimensions of the COVID-19 response in Chile and Paraguay. Our analysis, examples, and recommendations can contribute to the ongoing debates and learnings about how to strengthen policy and programming decisions and to the exploration of the conceptual framework put forward in Chap. 1. We know that the degree to which the COVID-19 pandemic, or any other outbreak or pandemic, continues to affect us greatly depends on the way each one of us behaves, interacts with our environments, especially wild animals, and interacts with each other. The actions and behaviors we decide to adopt, particularly as a result of communication and community engagement actions that are informed by context, trust, credibility, and rights, among other issues, will make a great difference in determining how successful we are in preventing and/or responding to the spread of COVID-19 and of any other viruses.

Disclaimer The views expressed in this chapter are those of the authors and do not represent the official position of UNICEF.

References

ADN Digital. (2020). *Gastronómicos desafían al gobierno y dicen que volverán a encender el fuego desde el lunes 25, mientras Mazzoleni apela a la conciencia del gremio*. Author.

Araya, A. (2020). *Expertos en comunicacion califican de ambivalente y deficitario el discurso del gobierno ante el Covid-19*. Universidad de Santiago de Chile Noticias. Retrieved from https://

www.usach.cl/news/expertos-comunicacion-califican-ambivalente-y-deficitario-discurso-del-gobierno-ante-covid-19

BBC. (2020). Coronavirus: Chile protesters clash with police over lockdown. *BBC News*.

Bicchieri, C. (2017). *Norms in the Wild*. Oxford University Press.

Boswell, T. (2017). *Tereré: Yerba mate and social practice in Paraguay*. The International Scholar (theintlscholar.com).

Carneri, S., & Politi, D. (2021, March 11). Indignación en Paraguay: la corrupción y el aumento de casos de la COVID-19 generan protestas. *The New York Times*. Spanish online edition.

Carnieri, S. and D. Politi. 2021. ´´Rage Spreads in Paraguay as Virus Surges, Exposing Corruption´´. *The New York Times*, March 11, 2021. Accessed on September 30th 2021.

Gerber, M., Cuadrado, C., Figueiredo, A., Crispi, F., Jiménez-Moya, G., & Andrade, V. (2021). Taking care of each other: How can we increase compliance with personal protective measures during the COVID-19 pandemic in Chile? *Political Psychology, 42*(5), 863–880. https://doi.org/10.1111/pops.12770

Gladwell, M. (2000). *The tipping point: How little things can make a big difference*. Little, Brown.

Gobierno de Chile. *Cifras Oficiales Covid-19*. Gob.cl - Cifras Oficiales. Retrieved from www.gob.cl

Goni, U., & Costa, W. (2020). Uruguay and Paraguay buck Latin America coronavirus trend. *The Guardian*.

Johns Hopkins University. (2021). *COVID-19 map*. Johns Hopkins Coronavirus Resource Center. Retrieved from https://coronavirus.jhu.edu/

La Nación. (2020). Salud confirma 29 nuevos casos de COVID-19, entre ellos 5 sin nexo. *La Nación*. Retrieved from www.lanacion.com.py

Martínez, M., Cuadrado, C., Goyenechea, M., Fica, D., & Peña, S. (2020). Chile frente al SARS-coV-2: Pandemia en medio del conflicto social. *Revista Chilena de Salud Pública, Special issue: "Virus y Sociedad: Hacer de la Tragedia social una Oportunidad de Cambios"*, 50–67.

Ministerio de Salud y Bienestar Social de Paraguay. (2020). *COVID-19 y la nueva forma de tomar mate*. Author. Retrieved from www.mspbs.gov.py

Miranda, B. (2020). *Las razones por las que Mañalich perdió la "batalla de Santiago": movilidad descontrolada y pérdida de la trazabilidad*. Centro de Investigación Periodística (CIPER). Retrieved from https://www.ciperchile.cl/2020/06/16/las-razones-por-las-que-manalich-perdio-la-batalla-de-santiago-movilidad-descontrolada-y-perdida-de-la-trazabilidad/

Mody, B. (1991). *Designing messages for development communication*. Sage Publications.

Reinharz, S. (1983). Experiential analysis: A contribution to feminist research. In G. Bowles & R. Duelli Klein (Eds.), *Theories of women's studies* (pp. 162–188). Routledge & Kegan Paul.

Rosenberg, T. (2011). *Join the club: How peer pressure can transform the world*. Norton.

Siegrist, M., & Zingg, A. (2014). The role of public trust during pandemics: Implications for crisis communication. *European Psychologist, 9*(1), 23. https://doi.org/10.1027/1016-9040/a000169

The Guardian. 2020. Uruguay and Paraguay buck Latin America coronavirus trend. Coronavirus. *The Guardian*. https://www.theguardian.com/world/2020/jun/25/uruguay-and-paraguay-buck-latin-america-coronavirus-trend (Accessed on September 30th, 2021).

Treader, V. (2020). *Paraguay, Uruguay y Costa Rica a la vanguardia de la lucha contra COVID-19*. Deutsche Welle America Latina. Retrieved from https://p.dw.com/p/3cYbO

UNICEF Paraguay. (2020). *National survey on the impact of COVID-19 on children in Paraguay*. UNICEF Paraguay, Asuncion.

Valcarcel, B., Avilez, J. L., Smith Torres-Roman, J., Poterico, J., Bazalar-Palacios, J., & La Vecchia, C. (2020). The effect of early stage public health policies in the transmission of Covid-19 in South American countries. *Revista Panamericana de Salud Pública, 44*, 1–7.

World Health Organization. (2020). *COVID-19 strategic preparedness and response plan: Operational planning guidelines to support country preparedness and response*. Author. covid-19-sprp-unct-guidelines.pdf (who.int).

Chapter 9
Communication and Community Engagement to Contain Disease Outbreaks and Improve Well-Being: Rohingya Refugee Response, Bangladesh

Neha Kapil, Aarunima Bhatnagar, Mohammad Alamgir, Ataul Gani Osmani, Mamunul Haque, and Sheikh Masudur Rahman

Contents

Introduction

Between August 2017 and February 2018, approximately 675,000 Rohingyas,[1] mainly women, children, and the elderly, crossed into the southern coastal district of Cox's Bazar (CXB), Bangladesh, fleeing violence and persecution in Myanmar. Combined with previous settlements of an estimated 215,000[2] registered and

[1] UNHCR (n.d.), Operational Dashboard on Myanmar Refugees. Accessed 20.05.2021.

[2] Numbers vary according to source and method of calculation. UNHCR estimates from 2020 have been utilized in this manuscript.

N. Kapil (✉)
UNICEF Middle East & North Africa Regional Office, Amman, Jordan
e-mail: nkapil@unicef.org

A. Bhatnagar
UNICEF, Baghdad, Iraq

M. Alamgir · A. G. Osmani
Field Office, UNICEF, Cox's Bazar, Bangladesh

M. Haque · S. M. Rahman
UNICEF, Dhaka, Bangladesh

E. Manoncourt et al. (eds.), *Communication and Community Engagement in Disease Outbreaks*, https://doi.org/10.1007/978-3-030-92296-2_9

unregistered Rohingyas in CXB, this situation grew very rapidly into one of the largest and most complex global refugee crises in recent years. Key priorities for national and international humanitarian responders working under the auspices of the Government of Bangladesh (GoB) included meeting the shelter, health, nutrition, water, sanitation, protection, and education rights of the refugees; mitigating disease and environmental risks; alleviating suffering; restoring dignity; and diffusing social tensions among the newly arrived and previously settled Rohingyas, as well as the host Bangladeshi communities.

Cox's Bazar, Bangladesh

The 2017 influx of the Rohingyas exacerbated the preexisting developmental challenges in CXB. This southeastern coastal district of the country, bordering Myanmar, has been low performing for decades. Low investments and recurring natural disasters such as cyclones have limited CXB's development, and it is considered as "lagging behind" national averages. A significant majority (78.5%) of CXB's 2.2 million population[3] is rural, and most communities live in hard-to-reach, underserved areas. Approximately 33% of the population lives below the poverty line compared to the national average of 31.5% (Ibid). The primary means of livelihood are agriculture, fishing, and the informal sector. Almost 12% (11.8%) of households do not have access to toilets and practice open defecation, compared to the national average of 7.7% (Ibid). Use of basic sanitation services is 42.6% compared to the national average of 64.4% (UNICEF and BBS, MICS, 2019). Institutional newborn deliveries in the district at 29.2% lie well below the national average of 53.4%; postnatal care for newborns and mothers at 39% and 37% is also below national averages of 66.7% and 65.3% respectively (UNICEF and BBS, MICS, 2019). Primary school age completion rates stand at 73.6% compared with the national figures of 80.6% (Ibid). The district also has high food insecurity and a poor nutritional status (UN, Cox's Bazar District Development Plan, 2019). CXB is socio-culturally diverse. Besides Bangla, much of the district's population speaks Chittagonian which is linguistically similar with Rohingya language and has facilitated communication between host and refugee communities. While most Bangladeshis in CXB are Sunni Muslims, minority religious groups also co-exist: the Hindus at approximately 4% of the population, followed by Buddhists at an estimated 2%. Despite the diversity, the district is culturally and religiously conservative compared to the rest of Bangladesh (Rashid, 2011). Bangladesh, overall, is a country of high religiosity, and religious leaders, institutions, and education are integral to public opinion, shape the values and beliefs of communities (Asia Foundation, 2015), and often are more trusted and influential than political actors (Marshall, 2015). The deep influence of religion in CXB has underscored advocacy with local Bangladeshi Islamic

[3] World Bank (2016), Bangladesh 2011 Census.

leaders to reach and engage the local host communities to support the delivery of services to the Rohingyas and promote social cohesion.

Due to porous borders with Myanmar, the Rohingyas have been crossing into CXB in small numbers since the 1970s, and for the past two decades, smaller-sized camps authorized by the government and managed by UN agencies have been in existence within the district.[4] The sudden influx of the Rohingyas in 2017, especially in large numbers, severely strained the resources available for the district, affected economic opportunities for the locals, and increased social tensions. It also had a major environmental impact with the erosion of large tracts of reserved forest area which provided cover to the inner areas of the district from cyclones and flooding (UN, Cox's Bazar District Development Plan, 2019). The district's development status, geography, and socio-political context have led many agencies such as UNICEF to establish programs and engage with local officials since the 1990s to accelerate development outcomes for local communities, including within the smaller, previously established Rohingya camps. These programs and previous relationships with local partners have been central to establishing and scaling up rapid responses with the massive influx of the Rohingyas between 2017 and 2018.

Rohingya Influx Situational Assessments

Multisectoral assessments that were conducted within weeks of the arrival of the Rohingyas in 2017 highlighted that arrivals had little knowledge of where and how to access services provided to them (ISCG Cox's Bazar, 2017), felt unheard, and were reluctant to file complaints (TWB, 2017), emphasizing the need for communication to promote life-saving services, risk-reduction behaviors, and mechanisms to provide feedback. Rapid, consistent, and complete information was needed on disease mitigation and care practices at household-level, utilization of relief commodities, and other protective behaviors. Communication was required to address risks, rumors, and misinformation; and promote healing, resilience, and social cohesion.

The early assessments also highlighted the importance of verbal communication, oral traditions, and interpersonal communication (IPC) for the Rohingyas (Internews & ETS, 2017). Illiteracy rates at 73% were high, with rates higher for women than men (Ibid). The Rohingya language is a spoken dialect with no written script. Only 17% males and 6% females of those who arrived in Bangladesh could speak, read, or understand basic Myanmar (TWB, 2017). With five major languages and dialects in use within the camps—Rohingya, English, Myanmar, Bangla, Chittagonian—the Rohingyas faced barriers in communicating with humanitarian responders (Ibid). Visual literacy was poor. Developing interpersonal communication (IPC) training tools and materials became a challenge. In addition, the use of digital technologies

---

[4] UNHCR (2017). This includes approximately 74,000 Rohingyas who crossed into CXB in mid-late 2016.

for rapid access to new information and real-time monitoring was complicated by limitations on using national SIM cards, mobile phones, and internet usage within the camps as per government regulations.[5]

Literature Review

Findings from a rapid literature review of the Rohingyas in Myanmar carried out by the Institute of Development Studies (IDS), Sussex University through the Social Sciences in Humanitarian Action Platform (SSHAP)[6] for UNICEF in late 2017 provided deeper insights to understand Rohingya culture and context before exodus. The Rohingyas have been historically and chronically underserved with severe restrictions on rights to identity[7] and livelihoods, movement and mobility, access to services, and political participation. The Rohingyas are Sunni Muslims (Ripoll, 2017). Religious life plays an important role in Rohingya culture; *imams* (Islamic religious leaders), *mullahs* (Islamic statesmen/heads of mosques), and *maulvis* (heads of madrassas) hold positions of influence, authority, and trust within their communities (Ibid) and are important stakeholders to consider in service outreach and social change efforts. While there are no significant social distinctions among the Rohingyas, gender is a crucial differentiator, and there are entrenched gender norms that define rigid roles for the sexes particularly female.[8] In Myanmar, Rohingyas practiced *purdah* (veiling of women's faces) and gender segregation, limiting women's engagement in earning livelihoods and public life (Ripoll, 2017). This has been brought into sharp contrast in the camps where females, a significant proportion of the arrivals, have had to engage in work outside the home, become breadwinners and step into public spaces. This has reportedly been one driver of increased incidents of reported threats, gender-based violence (GBV) and harassment. Marriage is an important milestone and provides security for women. Child marriage and polygamy were reported as increasing when in Myanmar but have accelerated after the influx due to lower numbers of men, safety concerns and economic difficulties in the camps (Ibid), implying increased vulnerabilities and risks for young girls. After marriage, a woman becomes the responsibility of the husband's family, and her mother-in-law plays an important role in guiding behavior for health, childcare, and other gendered tasks (Ibid). These insights have been crucial to understanding how to approach and engage women and girls of all ages in the response.

[5] The ban on use of internet was lifted as of 28.08.2020 (Dhaka Tribune, 2020).

[6] https://www.socialscienceinaction.org/.

[7] The Rohingyas are officially stateless. Human Rights Watch (2018).

[8] Some minor differences exist based on education, income levels, and age (Ripoll, 2017).

Rohingya Health Beliefs and Practices

Rohingya communities have been beset with poor health outcomes due to previous lack of access to formal health and education services while in Myanmar or, currently, due to physical conditions and overcrowding within the camps. The literature review highlighted that beliefs around health have been conditioned by the lack of access, unaffordability, and experiences of discrimination in Myanmar. There has been a high reliance on home and herbal remedies and alternative health providers such as traditional healers, herbalists, and faith healers. Disease and health are linked with spirituality and religion; and difficulties, disability, malnutrition, mental health issues are attributed to *jinns* (spirits) or the evil eye (Ibid). These beliefs have led to rumors, myths, and misinformation during, for example, diphtheria and acute watery diarrhea (AWD)/cholera outbreaks in the early days following the influx. A qualitative assessment conducted by the US Centers for Disease Control and Prevention (CDC), UNICEF, and WHO in early 2018 following diphtheria outbreaks in late 2017 found that community members reported using traditional treatments of gargling with hot water followed by an ingestion of chili-paste and salt mixture when they suspected having contracted diphtheria. Complex beliefs around vaccinations emerged, including one that vaccination led to a conversion into Christianity (Jalloh et al., 2019). A UNICEF and Innovations in Poverty Action (IPA) Knowledge, Attitudes, Practices and Behaviors (KAPB) Baseline Study in 2018 highlighted that while knowledge of vaccinations was high at the time of data collection, misconceptions of negative impacts persisted (UNICEF and IPA, KAPB Baseline, 2018).

Response

Humanitarian response in early phases focused on establishing essential services and supply chains to provide food, shelter, clean water, sanitation, and prevent disease outbreaks. Efforts to systematically reach, inform, consult, and engage communities to access services, reduce health risks, and practice life-saving behaviors were more limited. To address this, partners with expertise or experience in communication and community engagement (CCE) such as BBC Media Action (BBCMA), Johns Hopkins Center for Communication Programs (CCP), the Bangladeshi non-governmental organization BRAC, and Islamic Foundation Bangladesh (IFB) under the Ministry of Religious Affairs (MoRA), were swiftly mobilized by UNICEF to support this work. Prompted by AWD, measles and diphtheria outbreaks in the camps in the early months after the influx and, working through a previously convened "Communicating with Communities" Working

Group (CwC WG),[9] a promotional package of priority household healthcare behaviors and prevention practices was finalized in consultation with sectors.[10] Simultaneously, numerous platforms were developed for community mobilization, radio programming, stakeholder engagement, and community feedback, to promote these practices and improve accountability. The establishment of these multiple community engagement platforms was undergirded by evidence gathered through on-ground qualitative and quantitative assessments. These were initially conducted rapidly to generate behavioral insights, and later as the situation stabilized, through more rigorous methodologies, for representativeness. Information was triangulated from multiple sources including sector-specific needs assessments, partner reports, available but limited literature, and conceptual frameworks commonly utilized from the social and behavioral sciences to guide efforts.[11] Between 2017 and 2019, these platforms were utilized to roll out 22 multi-level campaigns. Starting with prevention and control of AWD, measles, dengue, diphtheria, and varicella, and promotion of vaccinations (e.g., cholera, polio, measles), these platforms helped foster credibility and trust among affected populations. Over time, they were leveraged to support wider education, protection, and nutrition goals; and prepare and respond to seasonal cyclones and natural disasters.

Community Mobilization

Drawing from UNICEF's global experiences in disease prevention programs on polio and ebola, as well as Bangladesh's successful immunization and community development programs, a multi-structured community mobilization platform was established in collaboration with BRAC for information outreach and dialogue. Called the "Community Mobilization Volunteer Network" (CMVn), this was a cornerstone of UNICEF's CCE response in the first 2 years after the influx. Composed of a trained, incentivized, and equipped frontline workforce of 1000 Rohingya volunteers, this platform had a routine coverage of 110,000 households (70% population equaling approximately 160,000 households in 2017/2018)[12] and full coverage across 34 camps during campaigns. In its first few months, the workforce covered 50,000 households and was scaled up to reach 110,000 in 2018. The workforce engaged with each household at least 25 times annually to disseminate messages and materials, discuss risks, and demonstrate recommended behaviors.

---

[9] The CwC WG was convened by UNICEF and IOM in February 2017 following the November 2016 influx and the organization of a CwC Training by the national CwC partner platform in Bangladesh called Shongjog (http://www.shongjog.org.bd).

[10] For UNICEF, refers primarily to health; nutrition; water sanitation, and hygiene (WASH); protection; and education sectors.

[11] For example, Social Ecological Model, Health Belief Model, and Diffusion of Innovations.

[12] Currently the figure is about 188,000 households as per UNHCR Operational Dashboard. Last accessed 20.12.20.

From the start, workforce planning and management were routinely challenged by low literacy, language constraints, threats to volunteer movement, high attrition, and shifting camp boundaries, for which corrective actions were taken. A four-tiered approach was designed: 10 Rohingya volunteers, each assigned around 100 households with at least contact per fortnight, were supervised by one on-ground Bangladeshi mobilization manager who was literate, spoke Chittagonian and was from the local host community; 100 of whom were in turn managed by 30 qualified project supervisors attached to 11 field offices. Five officers and management personnel monitored progress through monthly action plans. Incentives, aligned to the overall response guidelines, were provided to retain volunteers. Given the strong gender dimensions, and to promote the empowerment of women, females were given preference during recruitment. Approximately 85% of the workforce was female; and a reserve of trained candidates was maintained to manage attrition. To support the movement of the workforce, particularly female, advocacy with camp leaders (*majhis* and *imams*) was conducted for support from male community members. Capacities of camp stakeholders were built around "Prevention of Sexual Exploitation and Abuse (PSEA)", referral pathways, and gender dimensions of community engagement. Household assignment was done using geo-spatial mapping and randomized design, and volunteers were tagged which allowed for early identification and reassignment with changing camp boundaries. Workforce coordination mechanisms were created, and quality was assured through spots checks and joint visits for monitoring workforce performance.

A strong emphasis was placed on workforce capacity development. In partnership with CCP, regular and iterative training was incorporated in the project design based on training-needs assessments. This informed the development of a contextualized IPC training package combining adult-learning approaches for a low literacy audience. The content focused on key household care practices for health, disease prevention and well-being, and emphasized listening, discussion, empathy, and trust-building. The package, digitized for use in phones, included modules in Bangla to train managers who cascaded training to Rohingya volunteers in Chittagonian and Rohingya. To ensure consistency across the response, the package was rolled out to 260 master-trainers from partner organizations across the response architecture. To foster acceptability, training tools and audio-visual materials were developed in Chittagonian and Rohingya languages, using participatory approaches and joint analyses with the Rohingyas as co-producers and artists. They were distributed among CMVn managers through offline mobile applications and SD cards for smart- and lower-end feature-phones to ensure effective utilization. Post-training assessments and routine monitoring indicated that master-trainers and field-based CMVs found the trainings practical, engaging, and relevant. Tools and techniques were accepted among community members. Offline versions of the tools and materials improved access and reduced the load of carrying heavy print materials across the hilly terrains of the camps. Involving Rohingya communities in production helped build trust, appeal, understanding, and acceptance of the materials. Featuring local opinion and religious leaders in audio-visuals enabled difficult and sensitive discussions on topics such as child marriage and child protection. The tools and materials have also been adapted for use in host communities (Ergül, 2020a).

Upon its establishment, the workforce became one of the largest and most systematic multi-sectoral CCE platforms for rapid access to families across the 34 camps particularly during high-intensity campaigns on outbreak prevention and cyclone preparedness. It featured as an integral resource of the "Risk Communications Taskforce" under Health and CwC sectors comprising over 30 agencies. Health campaigns also included promotional efforts by an additional 300 Community Health Workers (CHWs) under the Health Sector and approximately 500 Hygiene Promoters (HPs) from the WASH sector who were semi-skilled and trained solely on health counseling and WASH promotion respectively. Together the CMVs, CHWs, and HPs supported local bottleneck analyses and micro-planning to target and coordinate outreach and engagement efforts and, followed up with families on immunization status and non-compliance, sometimes modeling vaccinations themselves. The efficacy of awareness-raising and mobilization efforts has been recognized by the health sector as one of the key drivers of the success of vaccination campaigns. Government reports have highlighted for instance that between October 2017 and December 2018, four oral cholera vaccination (OCV) campaigns achieved 106%, 109%, 89%, and 111% coverage rates respectively.[13] In the 2 years, no major or large-scale outbreaks were noted, and caseload ratios at peak, were reportedly less than 5% of the population.[14]

The role and contribution of the CMVn has also been reflected in formal and informal sector assessments and monitoring. For example, sector monitoring of "Nutrition Action Week (NAW)", March 2019 (Nutrition Action Week, 2019) highlighted that most parents knew of NAW through volunteers, of whom the CMVs were the majority; and over 84% of the "Infant and Young Child Feeding (IYCF)" messages were disseminated through them. Other key sources of information included mobile and mosque-based *miking* (microphone announcements) as well as information provided by *majhis* (camp leaders) who were in turn engaged and oriented by CMVs and CHVs. During cyclone warnings, CMVs assessed needs and damages to facilitate sector support. Until June 2019, 105 potential disaster incidents were avoided following information provided by the volunteers.[15] Routine monitoring, anecdotal evidence, and occasional threats to volunteers to stop work suggested that CMVs were becoming trusted sources of information and influence within the camps.

Maintaining a large-scale human resource intensive network is costly. The early advocacy for and availability of resources was a key determinant in establishing and scaling up the CMVn rapidly. Over time, planning for the continuity of this platform

---

[13] Vandenent et al. (2019). ASCODD Presentation.

[14] According to WHO (2018) specific disease reports (https://www.who.int/docs/default-source/searo/bangladesh/bangladesh%2D%2D-rohingya-crisis%2D%2D-pdf-reports/public-health-situation-analysis-may-2018.pdf?Status=Temp&sfvrsn=9a280761_2). A seroprevalence study is currently underway to determine this as indicated by the Health Sector Coordinator, CXB. 20.12.20.

[15] Ergül, (2020b), extracted from an interview with BRAC.

became essential as the crisis matured and stabilized because there was (and continues to be) no singular national organization or institutional system in the country that oversees CCE/SBCC to whom such a platform could gradually be handed over to, unlike in the health, education or water sanitation sectors. Initial inflows of funding helped in maintaining the CMVn for 2 years. By the end of 2019, there was a recognition of the slowdown in funding. Corresponding programmatic shifts and discussions were initiated to integrate the CMVn into sectoral workforces over the next few years, particularly into the health sector, that had received long-term structural funding for humanitarian-to-development programming transition. This was considered a suitable exit strategy that would, at the same time, enable the trained volunteers to continue earning livelihoods, build their skills further in specific sectoral areas for focused support to their peers, and improve their credentials in the informal job market.

Stakeholder Engagement

To augment community mobilization, over 5000 key community stakeholders including 4500 Rohingya religious leaders, 100 *hafezas* (female Islamic scholars), and others such as *majhis*, traditional healers and midwives were mobilized, oriented, and engaged over the 2 years through IFB and local partners. Religious and community leaders however are rarely a homogenous group and can be divided on social issues (Ergul, 2020d). Reaching and involving Rohingya religious leaders in response efforts was thus initially challenged by suspicion and misperceptions of the responders' agendas. This was addressed by leveraging UNICEF's national partnership with IFB and its vast network of local *imams* in the district to network and build trust with Rohingya *imams*. As relationships grew stronger and acceptability for supporting campaigns increased, orientation materials were developed to strengthen Rohingya *imams*' own understanding of disease, health, and well-being. Training sessions on social and behavior change were also provided to the *imams*, *hafezas*, and *majhis*, who subsequently supported message dissemination, promoted desired behaviors, particularly for vaccination, and fostered social cohesion between Rohingya communities and the local host population though Friday *khutba* (sermons), mosque announcements, and community dialogue.

Radio Programming

Radio is an important medium in the remote and coastal regions of Bangladesh such as CXB, used especially for early warning on cyclones and tropical storms. Given the importance of oral communication for Rohingyas, outreach by radio was identified early in the response as a low-cost supplementary means to rapidly disseminate information on disease risk mitigation practices in real-time to both host and

Rohingya communities. Radio was utilized also for host communities to dispel misconceptions about the Rohingyas; re-frame narratives of the situation to de-escalate tensions; and assure the local population of the continued attention to their developmental challenges and needs by district authorities and humanitarian agencies. Educational and interactive discussion programs and call-in shows such as *Betar Sanglap* (Radio Dialogue), *Begunnur Lai* (For All), and *Shishur Hashi* (Child's Laugh) were produced in collaboration with Bangladesh Betar (100.8 FM) the national radio under the Bangladesh Ministry of Information (MoI), and Community Radio Station "Naf" (99.2 FM) operated by the civil society organization ACLAB, with the technical support of BBCMA. While meant for the host population, they included issues and topics pertinent to the Rohingya communities and focused on grievances with the influx, promotion of disease control efforts including vaccination campaigns, as well as services available to both host and Rohingya communities. During the vaccination drives, repeated radio announcements, sometimes 10–12 times a day, served as reminders of vaccination points, and provided accurate information to quell rumors.[16]

Messaging through radio-based programming reached an estimated 1.29 million people (ACAPs, 2020) regularly within CXB. The use of radio, however, came with its own challenges, key of which were: low signal strength within the hilly terrains of the camps, the Rohingya communities' limited access to radio sets, and the one-way nature of communication. To address the issue of signal strength and drawing upon its long-standing partnership with MoI, UNICEF along with other partners advocated at the national level for the establishment of additional antennas to improve signal strength.[17] To improve access, 3,000 wind-up radio sets were distributed by UNICEF at key project locations and community meeting points, however proved insufficient to meet the needs at scale. Recognizing this, the International Organization for Migration (IOM) procured 60,000 radio sets for distribution at the household level. Until 2019, 32,445 households had direct access to radio sets (ISCG, 2019). In addition, programs were stored on portable storage or other mobile devices in offline formats and played back to community groups. To foster active listening and interactivity, UNICEF and CwC WG partners established radio listening groups with 12,028 participants reached by 752 radio-listening sessions, and 13,000 participants who accessed radio programs through narrowcasting (Ibid). Of these, UNICEF, in collaboration with local partners, supported 254 radio clubs within the camps and host communities to engage youth and adolescent boys and girls on health and well-being and build their capacities as agents of change for recommended behaviors.[18] To ensure the participation of girls, who would otherwise not be permitted to join the clubs, gender segregated sessions were held, led by female facilitators from partner NGOs.

[16] Ergül, (2020c), extracted from an interview with a partner.

[17] As of December 2020, this is under consideration by Bangladesh Betar as confirmed by UNICEF C4D team in Cox's Bazaar.

[18] Ergül (2020c), extracted from an interview with a partner.

The impact of radio programming has not been evaluated. However, a radio listenership assessment[19] conducted as recently as October 2020 revealed that 87% of respondents in host communities and Rohingya camps listen to radio programmes either through radio sets or feature phones, most tuning to Bangladesh Betar channels. Of these, 41.51% Rohingyas and 47% Bangladeshis listen to radio programmes daily. Respondents reported listening most to the three magazine programs *Jiboner Jonno*[20] and *Begguner Lai* from Betar, and *Shishur Hashi* from Radio Naf that have been covering Rohingya issues since 2017 highlighting the positive impact these programs have had. A qualitative study by BBCMA for UNICEF earlier in 2018 highlighted that respondents found the information provided by the programs while not entirely new, to be trustworthy, relevant, and useful to them (UNICEF and BBC Media Action, 2018).

Community Feedback and Response Mechanism

Drawing from UNICEF's (n.d.) "Core Commitments to Children",[21] as well as Grand Bargain (n.d.)[22] and World Humanitarian Summit (n.d.)[23] commitments on "Accountability to Affected Populations (AAP)," a platform for systematically gathering community feedback on response services and addressing queries was created. Fourteen Information and Feedback Centers (IFCs) were established in collaboration with local non-governmental partners PULSE, BITA, and ACLAB. The IFCs are physical facilities located at strategic points within the camps and serve as "one-stop shops" for community members to register grievances, gather information, and obtain referrals for services. IFCs receive and respond to these complaints, feedback, and queries (CFQs), and promote practices for community health and social well-being. IFCs are managed by in-facility Information Service Providers (ISPs) who are trained on IPC, feedback provision, and service referrals including for more complex gender issues as they pertain to PSEA. IFCs also include a supplementary and trained cadre of 320 mobile volunteers, comprising females (popularly known as *model mothers*) and youth, from the Rohingya communities. CFQs are recorded in logbooks, responded to daily, and digitized anonymously for aggregation through an online platform for trends analyses and forecasting.

In 2018, to strengthen the linkage between humanitarian and development programming and improve accountability of local government initiatives, UNICEF established one IFC each in four *upazilas* (sub-districts) of CXB to gather feedback and grievances from host communities, thereby bringing the total up to 18 IFCs. In

[19] RAPID Study (2020), Draft/Unpublished.

[20] National level program based on UNICEF Facts for Life publication.

[21] https://www.unicef.org/emergencies/core-commitments-children.

[22] https://interagencystandingcommittee.org/grand-bargain.

[23] https://agendaforhumanity.org/summit.html.

addition, the IFCs' scope of work was enhanced to include a stronger outreach to children and people living with disabilities, one of the most vulnerable and marginalized groups within the camps. For this, operating procedures were revised, and specific inclusive and educational materials[24] were designed and disseminated through ISPs and model mothers. From October 2017, when the first IFC was founded, to December 2019, approximately 165,000 cases of CFQs were filed, majority of which related to health issues and were resolved at the camp-level itself.[25]

Besides its own investments in establishing IFCs, UNICEF led the *Information Hub (IH) Sub-Working Group* under the larger CwC WG, to support the activation of 85 other information hubs, many of which focused on more specialized services such as shelter. Data gathered from the hubs informed the planning and the implementation of health and other campaigns. A publicly available online dashboard[26] was designed by UNICEF as part of the feedback and response mechanism, and a set of common Standard Operating Procedures (SOPs) and training tools were developed for inter-agency referrals and meta-data analysis to guide preparedness and response.

A key challenge that emerged after the establishment of the IFCs was low awareness and uptake of such a service in respective catchment areas. Rohingyas, with their history of being ignored, underserved, and marginalized, did not see the relevance and utility of such a service. The outreach workforce of the IFCs, model mothers and youth volunteers, proved invaluable here in promoting the IFCs and creating an initial pull of those who had grievances, needed service referrals, or were seeking information. Responding quickly and accurately became necessary not only to ensure quality of service but also to build reputation and recognition. For this, the monitoring of the IFCs was intensive in the first year of operation. As relevance and reputation improved, GBV complaints started filtering in, triggering a need to improve response protocols and service referrals. In close collaboration with the Protection Sector, cases of GBV and PSEA were addressed based on the nature of the complaint and a clear protocol. All complaints were referred to the Protection Sector with adherence to strict confidentiality and privacy. As complaints were made primarily by women, IFCs were re-modeled to include "private" rooms or areas with female-only service providers, and referrals were followed up by the female ISP in the IFC. This was a critical step in closing the "feedback loop" which emerged as another challenge as recorded cases of CFQs increased. A UNICEF rapid internal assessment (UNICEF Community Accountability Study, Internal Document, 2019) found that 93% of the issues recorded in the IFCs linked primarily to service referrals and were resolved within the same day at camp-level. However, gaps and delays in closing feedback loops at institutional and overall response levels

[24] For example, audio-visual materials from the Meena Communication Initiative were dubbed in Rohingya and played in the camps.

[25] A rapid internal assessment in mid-2019 by UNICEF found that up to 93% recorded cases were resolved at camp level itself.

[26] http://ifc.unicefbangladesh.org/2/.

persisted. Data needed to be disseminated more widely to identify trends in community needs and improve services. To this end, training sessions for IH Sub-Working Group members were held to standardize feedback cycles, and referral systems on the ground were strengthened by improving ties with service centers. Agencies operating the hubs, along with camp authorities, made joint visits to ensure effective monitoring and coordination and disseminated data more widely. These measures helped improve services and, in 2019, during the campaigns for AWD, measles and nutrition, joint mission teams observed the information hubs to be a source of information and referrals to health services.

In mid-2019, UNICEF, in partnership with Translators Without Borders (TWB, 2019a), conducted a rapid assessment of information hubs across the camps that highlighted their success in delivering life-saving information and serving as a credible service point for the Rohingyas to air grievances, provide feedback, and gather information. However, some language barriers were noted that lead to miscommunication (TWB, 2019b). To address this, the use of language glossaries and language training for field staff was accelerated. The 2019 Mid-term Review of the Joint Response Plan for Rohingya Humanitarian Crisis reaffirmed the role of information hubs highlighting that 59% of refugees (compared to 52% in 2018) knew how to make suggestions/complaints about the aid they received (Ground Truth Solutions (GTS), 2019). Among them, 27% made complaints with 66% of them being mostly satisfied with the response received (Ibid). Seventy-nine percent of households reported having no barriers to using feedback mechanisms (Multi-Sectoral Needs Assessment, 2019). With more than ten agencies currently utilizing a common system for sharing data, feedback loops have been improving, and there is evidence that humanitarian agencies and district authorities are making changes in the design of their programs based on community feedback and that information hubs are contributing to building an environment of credibility and trust in services.

Language, Mid-Media Outreach, Communication Supplies, and Material Dissemination

Language barriers were addressed through partnering with TWB and local groups to create language guides, multi-lingual glossaries and word banks, particularly around complex humanitarian response terminology, that were used for language training of field staff (Ergul, 2020e). Community mobilization, stakeholder engagement, and radio programming were augmented by regular distribution of locally designed and pretested educational materials, and communication supplies such as microphones and electronic tablets. Mid-media outreach included "miking" by mobile field staff and mosques within the Rohingya settlements. These proved invaluable and cost-effective for rapid and wide diffusion of messages on vaccination campaigns, in the immediate days following influx, and while some of the volunteer platforms were being established and scaled up. Other smaller scale initiatives included the use of interactive participatory theatre (IPT) performances with adolescents and community arts (wall paintings and murals) projects grounded in entertainment-education and creative arts approaches to promote healing, build confidence and cohesion, and foster ownership for localized action.

KAPB Surveys and Impact Assessment

To assess changes in Rohingya and host community knowledge, attitudes, practices, and behaviors, surveys were commissioned through IPA to collect baseline (UNICEF & IPA, 2018) and midline (UNICEF & IPA, 2019) data. Topics pertained to the promotional package of household care practices for health and well-being and included prevention of major diseases such as AWD, diarrhea, and pneumonia; vaccination; reproductive health and early childbearing; menstrual hygiene; newborn care; breastfeeding and complementary feeding; birth registration; hygiene and water safety; child protection with a focus on unaccompanied and separated children; child marriage; gender-based violence; HIV/AIDS; and trusted sources of information. The baseline included both qualitative and quantitative methods, with a two-stage randomized cluster sampling utilized for the latter.

Impact Assessment

Using the opportunity of the surveys, and a planned endline study in 2020, UNICEF and IPA initiated an impact assessment component for the CMVn platform during the midline using experimental design to identify the direct impacts of the CMVn intervention on recipient households as well as the indirect spillover effects of the intervention on non-recipient households. The aim was to highlight the total effects of the community engagement intervention, as also assess changes among CMVs themselves which would give vital information to humanitarian responders in the long term on approaches to, and investments for, community engagement. The methodology for the midline included a randomized saturation design to study direct and spillover effects of the intervention on recipients and non-recipients. Comparability to the baseline, and ethical considerations were given a priority and methodology agreed upon before initiating this component. The experimental design was important because the CMVn intervention could impact neighbors as knowledge spreads through both primary and secondary diffusion. Blocks within camps were randomly assigned to saturation levels, where 0%, 50%, or 100% of households were contacted by the CMVn, without compromising the overall planned coverage (110,000 households) of the intervention. Over the course of the design of the study, challenges emerged in maintaining the saturation levels in the blocks (sub-divisions of camps) due to relocation and movement of refugees within camps, and increasing social tensions. For instance, and with the initial randomized sampling approach, the CMVn did not have the capacity to visit all households within some sub-blocks that required 100% saturation as specified by the experiment. These sub-blocks were dropped and added to a list of reserves that could be used to meet targets. This ensured that the CMVs could complete their targets without affecting the research design and ethics of humanitarian intervention outreach. Additionally, some households in the control group were mistakenly treated by the workforce. Such blocks were dropped from the study sample. To address the relocation of camps due to landslides and congestion, reserves were used to replace areas that were affected.

Unfortunately, the planned endline survey scheduled in 2020 could not be completed because of COVID-19 lockdowns. Were an endline to be conducted in 2021, delays in gathering data at this later time will compromise the impact assessment component linked to the CMVn as workforce numbers were gradually reduced in 2020. Despite this setback, the responses to the methodological challenges, and outcomes of adjustments to the experimental component of the study to respond to the dynamic context, provide important lessons for future impact assessments in humanitarian contexts.

Findings[27]

Notwithstanding the failure to complete the experimental study, baseline (2018) and midline (2019) data comparisons showed between mixed to positive results with respect to changes in the KAPB of families over time. For example, knowledge and practice of vaccinations were quite similar from baseline to the midline. High percentages of respondents in camps and the host communities knew about vaccination and reasons for administration. However, awareness about how many times a child should get vaccinated by the age of 15 months varied across time (see Table 9.1).

About half of the camp and the host community respondents, in both the baseline and the midline, believed that their children under 2 had received all the necessary vaccinations. Vaccination of children at least once was high in the baseline and increased in the midline although there is variation in the number of vaccinations received (see Table 9.2).

Practices related to childbirth such as ante- and post-natal care and delivery were analyzed based on location of delivery of youngest child and were found to be significantly better for those that delivered their youngest child in Bangladesh compared to those that did in Myanmar over time. The incidence of home deliveries increased from baseline to midline. Parental knowledge about prenatal danger signs improved over time. For instance, 51% of the respondents in the camps and 60% in the host communities knew of the five maternal danger signs in the baseline.

[27] Summarized from UNICEF and IPA (2019).

Table 9.1 Knowledge of the number of times a child needs to get a vaccine before the age of 15 months

Midline			Baseline	
Number of times	Camps (%)	Host communities (%)	Camps (%)	Host communities (%)
Don't know	22.8	11.1	32.0	11.1
0	0.3	0.2	1.2	0.0
1	1.5	0.3	2.1	0.4
2	3.9	0.3	4.4	1.2
3	45.7	12.0	25.6	8.9
4	11.4	7.8	8.1	10.7
5	25.4	45.9	22.1	48.3
6	9.4	22.8	2.0	12.3
N Camp—2518			*N* Camp—2432	
N Host—665			*N* Host—740	

Source: UNICEF and IPA (2019), p. 111

Table 9.2 Number of vaccinations children received before the age of 15 months (*N* as Table 9.1)

Midline			Baseline	
Number of vaccinations	Camps (%)	Host communities (%)	Camps (%)	Host communities (%)
Don't know	0.6	1.6	6.1	4.6
0	0.4	0.3	1.0	0.8
1	13.0	3.8	10.8	2.8
2	18.1	6.3	16.4	5.7
3	37.9	18.3	36.5	15.2
4	14.6	18.8	14.2	21.9
5	10.9	31.9	12.0	33.7
6	5.2	20.7	2.8	15.4

Source: UNICEF and IPA (2019), p. 115

Knowledge among women was about 10 percentage points higher than among men in the camps and the host communities. In the midline, this increased to 66% in camps and 78% in the host communities, and on average, the knowledge level of women was almost 18 percentage points higher than of men in both camps and host communities. Knowledge of newborn care among Rohingya and the host communities improved over time. For instance, in the baseline, two-thirds of Rohingyas mentioned the need to dry and wrap a baby which increased to 84.3% in the midline. The percentage of respondents who mentioned the need for immediate breastfeeding increased from one-third to about half; however, more than 90% of respondents were still unaware of other practices such as delayed bathing.

Knowledge and practices for drinking water showed mixed changes from baseline to midline. Procurement of water from tube wells decreased in both camps and host communities, while perceptions and practice of water safety did not improve from baseline to the midline. Latrine use remained the same in the baseline and the midline; however, there were improvements reported in feces and garbage disposal practices. Handwashing with soap remained broadly consistent across the time periods and high (over 90%) for both Rohingya and host communities, with some improvements in knowledge of the need for handwashing before feeding a child. Findings related to diarrhea and diarrheal disease management remained consistent over the baseline and midline; however, gaps remained. For example, half of the respondents reporting giving a mixture of water and salt to children with diarrhea rather than oral saline.

Indicators for other areas also showed mixed results. For example, while literacy rates remained low across baseline and midline, educational aspirations improved substantially in the midline especially for women as compared to the baseline. Children's attendance in learning centers improved from the baseline to the midline. Knowledge of lost or unaccompanied children did not appear to change much from the baseline to midline, as did knowledge of menstrual hygiene practices. While there are some similar findings in the baseline and midline for GBV, there are also some notable differences in specific findings in relation to what got counted as abuse and on reporting.

Both baseline and midline show similar findings regarding sources of information and channels of communication. Most Rohingyas mentioned *majhis* and *masjid* (mosque) miking as a main source of information, and trust in this improved over time. The use of mobile phones increased over time, despite limitations on connectivity, and family and friends continued to play a role in disseminating information. The proportion of respondents who mentioned direct service from the CMVn, community leaders, and religious leaders fell from the baseline; however, in contrast, the use of face-to-face communication for critical information, with the same volunteers and stakeholders, increased from 78% of respondents in the baseline to 98%, across almost all respondents, in the midline. This contradiction highlighted, among other factors, that language issues persisted and "recognition" of the mobilization volunteers as providing a "service" was required. Awareness of available services in the community remained consistent across baseline and midline.

Follow-Up Actions

Information from the midline survey helped determine whether the CCE initiatives undertaken across the response were appropriate and effective, while also identifying changing needs and obstacles. Community mobilization was intensified through refresher training for the CMVn that incorporated revised content as a result. Health and nutrition messaging, dialogue, and referrals were simplified and strengthened. Communication materials and techniques were improved to include more interaction particularly from children. Linkages with disability and women-friendly centers were strengthened, and feedback from the IFCs was also examined more closely to identify further changes required. Installation of television sets in health centers was supported to improve information uptake given the low literacy levels. IPC training was also extended to other sectoral outreach workers such as CHWs and child support workers to bolster efforts by the CMVn.

Lessons Learned and Recommendations

A refugee crisis requires addressing not only health challenges and disease outbreaks, but also, and simultaneously, wider contextual issues and multi-sectoral rights deprivations. The systematic use of CCE in such humanitarian contexts is an evolving area of practice and study. Much of the easily accessible documented literature has focused either solely on public health emergencies such as the ebola and zika outbreaks[28] or on disaster responses.[29] At the time of the Rohingya influx, very few SOPs, technical guidance, and proven operational packages on CCE existed to guide early response to addressing a wide range of both health and non-health risks and challenges during a rapid-onset, large-scale, and complex refugee crisis. Case studies, examples of good practice, and lessons learned were also limited.

To contribute toward building evidence in this area, in 2019, UNICEF initiated the documentation of its CCE response in the first years after the influx. Seven institutional case studies, each detailing the distinct operational activities described previously, were developed and provide a robust set of lessons learned (Ergül, 2020a). These are synthesized and augmented to highlight the importance of: (1) engaging with broader humanitarian response architecture early on to integrate CCE approaches; (2) conducting rapid literature reviews and social research to understand the conditions, culture, and context of refugees in the location of their origin; (3) collecting behavioral data periodically to track progress and assess changes; (4) establishing partnerships swiftly to design and scale up multi-level, dialogical CCE platforms to address risks of disease outbreaks and promote life-saving practices, with an underlying goal of building acceptability of, and trust in, the response among refugees as they find themselves in a new environment and culture; (5) leveraging the trust in, and credibility of, these platforms over time to advance other sectoral goals for cost-efficiencies and effectiveness; (6) working with local organizations, and engaging both host and affected community members in response efforts to foster interaction, empathy, and understanding, improve social cohesion, and facilitate livelihoods; (7) mobilizing local and religious leaders to support sustained behavior change and refugee empowerment initiatives, albeit with careful consideration to ensure stakeholders do not resist social change; (8) promoting asset-based/positive narratives of refugees to bridge socio-political divides, restore dignity, reduce social tensions and improve cooperation, all essential to advance community health and well-being; (9) investing in girls' and women's training and empowerment to address entrenched gender norms and counter male-dominated

---

[28] For example, Gillespie et al. (2016).

[29] For example, Beggs (2018).

power structures that hinder uptake of desired household practices and services; (10) ensuring coordinated, consistent, and clear communication with affected communities across all platforms by all humanitarian responders, and establishing widely endorsed SOPs to do so; (11) fostering coordination among agencies that have established CCE volunteer workforces to rationalize workforce cadres and incentive systems, and avoid high cross-attrition, duplication, and misinformation; (12) conducting regular bottleneck analyses and micro-planning by issue (e.g., vaccinations or disaster preparedness) for focused action, ownership, and efficacy; (13) embedding iterative cycles of learning and training in program design to manage complexity, mitigate risks, and ensure relevance of efforts; and (14) collecting regular and protected feedback through face-to-face fixed and mobile mechanisms, and closing feedback loops at all (camp/institutional/sectoral/overall response) levels to address service gaps, rumors, and misinformation.

Recommendations

While ensuring that rights-based values and principles of community participation, voice, agency, and empowerment, along with AAP, remain central to CCE in any humanitarian context, three critical areas of consideration and action are suggested for those working in early response to a dynamic multi-sectoral refugee crisis:

1. *Rapidly integrate CCE into early response, leveraging initial disease prevention and outbreak communication efforts as a gateway to build CCE systems and strengthen a multi-dimensional response over time.* In a fast-evolving crisis where affected populations are on the move, and decisions are taken, and operations activated, within 24- to 48-h timeframes, time and timing are crucial factors, and speed is of the essence. In the early chaos and confusion that often follows a rapidly evolving refugee crisis of large scale, some of the "softer," more intangible areas such as information needs and communication with affected people can get lost or ignored in the midst of urgent and pressing needs of food, water, shelter, and protection. Humanitarian responders must ensure that CCE is also in focus in early response discussions and is evidence-based, coordinated, and inclusive, aiming to foster trust and dignity. This is crucial to prevent morbidity and mortality due to disease outbreaks that will likely follow due to inadequate living conditions, lack of access to preventive services and supplies, and inadequate family- and community-level risk-mitigation practices, the last where CCE is most urgently required. Over time, CCE assets can be leveraged to achieve wider sectoral outcomes for a comprehensive multi-dimensional and holistic response. Integrating CCE in response efforts from the start can pay dividends in the long-term by ensuring that: (1) the affected people are consulted and their needs assessed, from the beginning rather than as an afterthought, be it for health or other social challenges; (2) CCE strategies and packages are delivered alongside health and social services to build trust in the humanitarian

response and those delivering it; and (3) CCE components are included within overall humanitarian response architecture, and budgeted and resourced early on.

2. *Generate, diversify, and triangulate contextual and situational evidence:* Global, national, and institutional commitments to uphold human rights and minimum standards of emergency response provide the rationale and basis for action. Data, evidence, and feedback are required to guide the design and revision of these actions and cannot be emphasized enough especially in the context of a rapidly evolving multi-dimensional emergency. While rigorous research, especially to assess attribution, may be very challenging in the early days of response, it is imperative for responders working in the area of CCE to invest in gathering data rapidly even if this may not be representative initially. Diversity in approaches, flexibility in methodology, and triangulation of data from multiple sources is critical to develop approaches, test assumptions, and address design challenges. Rapid literature reviews and contextual assessments on refugee culture and conditions before exodus are crucial to inform responses. As responses mature and the lives of affected communities stabilize, more rigorous approaches are required with special emphasis on longitudinal data collection to measure behavioral and social changes. Besides KAPB surveys, CCE specialists should consider investing in other types of studies such as social norms research, rumor tracking, and feedback trends analyses. Qualitative methodologies can be used to capture more subtle shifts in power structures, relationships, and culture over time. The use of digital technologies should be leveraged to establish "real-time systems" to facilitate immediacy in process and performance data entry, access, and analysis. Experimental research, though challenging, is possible. It requires wide consultations to address methodological challenges, and very critically, it must ensure ethical considerations are not overlooked or compromised particularly in the delivery of humanitarian aid, including information and communication services, to those who are most affected.
3. *Plan for scale and sustainability:* During a large humanitarian crisis of a multidimensional nature, disease outbreaks, whether simultaneous or in succession, can rapidly overwhelm and exhaust existing national health and other sectoral systems, for which supplementary systems and platforms may need to be established and at scale. For refugees in camps particularly, achieving disease prevention and control targets at scale is often crucial due to crowded living conditions that could exacerbate the spread of infectious diseases. Correspondingly, responsive and at-scale CCE platforms become important for facilitating behavior change and improving accountability although they can be time-consuming and labor intensive to establish. To address the time lag between incidence of disease and availability of at-scale trained human resources for awareness-raising and widespread mobilization, solutions such as rapid procurement and distribution of supplies and materials, media programs and public service announcements, as well as digital and social media outreach can be utilized. These will create an initial groundswell of knowledge and uptake of desired behaviors and services. Maintaining all platforms for long-term social and behavior change however requires planning and advocacy. Without forecasting for and investing in the

relevance, stability, and longevity of these platforms, CCE efforts risk becoming ad hoc, reactive, disconnected, uncoordinated and ultimately, resource-heavy. Global, regional, and national-level humanitarian responders supporting CCE should seek to define a set of core standards, principles, and procedures around an operational package of proven CCE approaches and platforms that can be activated, scaled up, localized, and sustained within a sudden onset multi-sectoral refugee crisis or similar dynamic humanitarian context. This will: (1) reduce confusion and guesswork; (2) provide clear pathways for rapid, well-designed, coordinated, stable, and sensitive responses to both health and non-health issues; (3) enable fundraising for the long-term; and (4) most effectively utilize the power and potential of CCE to improve the health and well-being of populations affected by a refugee crisis.

Contributions and Acknowledgments The authors would like to acknowledge the following individuals and organizational partners, whose support was invaluable:

1. Hakan Ergul, Mohammed Ashraful Haque and Himali Kapil reviewed the manuscript. All the co-authors approved the final version of the manuscript.

Additionally, the individuals and partners listed below provided critical guidance, support, and contributions to the CCE response in CXB:

2. Gita Rani Das, Sayeeda Farhana, Yasmin Khan, Rizwan Nabin, Nasir Ateeq, Jon Bugge, Paryss Kouta, Nizamuddin Ahmed, Tobgye Tobgye, Naureen Naqvi, Umme Halima, Ambareen Khan, Mousumi Tripura, Mollah Mahmud, Didarul Alam, Sardar Arif-Uddin, Nana Garbrah-Aidoo, Farid Alam Khan, Parveen Azam, Shohely Sharmin, Michael Karmaker, Sohana Naznin, Yulia Widati, Balwinder Singh Chawla, Mukesh Prajapathi, ASM Mainul Hasan, Md. Golam Naser, Egmond Evers, Martin Worth, Juanita Vasquez Escallon, Carlos Acosta, Deepak Kumar Dey, Cheayoon Choo, Adam Tibe, Roots Bondowe, Maya Vandenent, Tania Sultana, Ehsan Ul-Haque, Bina D'Costa, Hakan Ergul, Edouard Beigbeder, Sheema Sengupta, Abdelkader Musse, Madhuri Banerjee, Jean Metenier, Naqibullah Safi, Sara Bordas Eddy, Shairose Mawji, Tomoo Hozumi, Veera Mendonca, Jean Gough, Viviane Steirteghem, and UNICEF Operations Team.

3. Partners include: MoI and MoRA, particularly Bangladesh Betar and the Islamic Foundation Bangladesh; RRRC; BRAC; PULSE; BITA; ACLAB/Radio Naf; SHED; CCP; IPA; IDS Sussex/SSHAP; Rain Barrel Communications, Drik, BBC Media Action, Translators Without Borders, IOM, and other members of the CWC WG. Financial support for this response package was received from Governments of Canada, Australia, Germany, Japan, the United Kingdom, the United States of America, and the European Union.

Disclaimer The views expressed in this report are those of the authors and do not necessarily represent the official position of UNICEF or the CwC WG in CXB.

References

Asia Foundation. (2015). *Religion and development in Bangladesh*. Author. Retrieved December 20, 2020, from https://asiafoundation.org/resources/pdfs/BGReligionandDevelopment.pdf

BBC Media Action Research and Learning Group. (2018). *Evaluating BBC Media Action's support to emergency radio programming to respond to the Rohingya crisis in Cox's Bazar, Bangladesh, UNICEF-funded project*. UNICEF. (Unpublished/Internal Report).

Beggs, J. C. (2018). Chapter 14 - Applications: Disaster communication and community engagement. In J. A. Horney (Ed.), *Disaster epidemiology* (pp. 163–169). Academic Press. https://doi.org/10.1016/B978-0-12-809318-4.00022-8. ISBN 9780128093184.

BBC Media Action (BBCMA) (2019) Common Service for Community Engagement & Accountability. (2019). *What contribution is the Common Service making to community engagement and accountability in the Rohingya response?* BBC Media Action.

Dhaka Tribune. (2020). 3G, 4G internet restored in Rohingya camps. *Dhaka Tribune*. Retrieved December 20, 2020, from https://www.dhakatribune.com/bangladesh/rohingya-crisis/2020/08/28/3g-4g-internet-restored-in-rohingya-camps

Ergül, H. (2020a). *Looking back to see forward: A case study collection on UNICEF's response to the Rohingya Refugee crisis*. UNICEF. Retrieved from https://www.unicef.org/bangladesh/en/reports/looking-back-see-forward

Ergül, H. (2020b). *Mobilizing for change: Strengthening engagement through community mobilization volunteers in Cox's Bazaar, Bangladesh*. UNICEF. Retrieved from https://www.unicef.org/bangladesh/en/reports/mobilizing-change

Ergül, H. (2020c). *Staying tuned: Radio programming for sustained behaviour change and accountability in Cox's Bazar, Bangladesh*. UNICEF. Retrieved from https://www.unicef.org/bangladesh/en/reports/staying-tuned

Ergül, H. (2020d). *The role of faith in the humanitarian response: Strengthening community participation and engagement through religious leaders in Rohingya Camps in Cox's Bazar*. UNICEF. Retrieved from https://www.unicef.org/bangladesh/en/reports/role-faith-humanitarian-response

Ergül, H. (2020e). *More than words: UNICEF's response to language barriers in Rohingya Refugee camps*. UNICEF.

Food Security Cluster. (2020). *ACAPs Cox's Bazar Upazila Analaysis*. Author. Retrieved December 20, 2020, from https://fscluster.org/coxs-bazar/document/acaps-coxs-bazar-upazila-profiles

Gillespie, A. M., Obregon, R., El Asawi, R., Richey, C., Manoncourt, E., Joshi, K., Naqvi, S., Pouye, A., Safi, N., Chitnis, K., & Quereshi, S. (2016). Social mobilization and community engagement central to the Ebola response in West Africa: Lessons for future public health emergencies. *Global Health: Science and Practice, 4*(4), 626–646. https://doi.org/10.9745/GHSP-D-16-00226

Ground Truth Solutions. (2019). *Rohingya feedback & relationships bulletins. Jun 2018, Dec 2018*. Author. Retrieved from https://reliefweb.int/report/bangladesh/bulletin-rohingya-feedback-and-relationships-june-2019

Human Rights Watch. (2018). *The plight of Rohingya Refugees from Myanmar*. Author. Retrieved from https://www.hrw.org/report/2018/08/05/bangladesh-not-my-country/plight-rohingya-refugees-myanmar

Inter Sector Coordination Group. (2018). *2019 Midterm review of Joint response plan for Rohingya humanitarian crisis*. SEG. Retrieved January 5, 2021, from https://www.humanitarianresponse.info/sites/www.humanitarianresponse.info/files/documents/files/2019_jrp_mid_term_review_final_for_circulation1_compressed.pdf

Inter Sector Coordination Group (ISCG). (2017). *Multi-sectoral rapid assessments-influx, Cox's Bazar*. Author. Retrieved December 18, 2020, from https://reliefweb.int/report/bangladesh/multi-sectoral-rapid-assessments-influx-makeshift-spontaneous-settlements-and-host

Inter Sector Coordination Group (ISCG). (2019). *'Situation report Rohingya refugee crisis', Cox's Bazar*. Author. Retrieved from https://reliefweb.int/sites/reliefweb.int/files/resources/sitrep_april_2019.pdf

Internews and Emergency Telecommunications Sector (ETS). (2017). *Information needs assessment, Cox's Bazar*. Author. Retrieved from https://internews.org/resource/information-needs-assessment-coxs-bazar-bangladesh

ISCG (2020). Joint Multi-Sector Needs Assessment (J-MSNA) Rohingya Refugees September 2019. Avaiable at https://www.humanitarianresponse.info/en/operations/bangladesh/document/coxs-bazar-joint-multi-sector-needs-assessment-msna-reportrohingya

Jalloh Mohamed, F., Bennett, S. D., Alam, D., Kouta, P., Lourenço, D., Alamgir, M., Feldstein, L. R., Ehlman, D. C., Abad, N., Kapil, N., Vandenent, M., Conklin, L., & Wolff, B. (2019). Rapid behavioral assessment of barriers and opportunities to improve vaccination coverage among displaced Rohingyas in Bangladesh, 2018. *Vaccine, 37*(6), 833–838. ISSN 0264-410X. Retrieved from https://www.sciencedirect.com/science/article/pii/S0264410X18317158?via%3Dihub

Marshall, K. (2015). *Faith and development in focus: Bangladesh*. World Faith Development Dialogue, Barkley Centre for Peace and World Affairs, Georgetown University.

Nutrition Action Week. (2019). Retrieved from https://public.tableau.com/profile/shami.shawal#!/vizhome/NAWRound3final/Dashboard1

Rashid, M. M. (2011). Shonglap: An innovation to break conservativeness and agent of change in rural Bangladesh Mohammed Mamun Rashid. *International NGO Journal, 6*(3), 86–90. https://doi.org/10.5897/NGOJ10.044. ISSN 1993–8225. Retrieved from http://www.academicjournals.org/INGOJ

Research and Policy Integration for Development (RAPID). (2020). *Radio listenership survey in Cox's Bazar District*. UNICEF and Bangladesh Betar, GoB. (Unpublished).

Ripoll, S. (2017). *Social and cultural factors shaping health and nutrition, wellbeing and protection of the Rohingya within a humanitarian context*. Social Science in Humanitarian Action. Retrieved from https://opendocs.ids.ac.uk/opendocs/handle/20.500.12413/13328

The Grand Bargain. (n.d.). Retrieved December 19, 2020, from https://interagencystandingcommittee.org/grand-bargain

Translators Without Borders (TWB). (2017). *Rohingya Zoban: rapid assessment of language barriers in the Cox's Bazar refugee response*. Author. Retrieved December 18, 2020, from https://www.arcgis.com/apps/Cascade/index.html?appid=683a58b07dba4db189297061b4f8cd40

Translators Without Borders (TWB). (2019a). *Information hubs assessment report May 2019*. Author.

Translators Without Borders (TWB). (2019b). *Bangladesh and Myanmar: Language needs across borders*. Author. Retrieved from https://translatorswithoutborders.org/myanmar

UN. (2019). *District development plan for Cox's Bazar*. Author. Retrieved from https://fscluster.org/rohingya_crisis/document/coxs-bazar-district-development-plan

UNHCR. (2017). *Rohingya influx strains camp resources in Bangladesh*. Author. Retrieved December 20, 2020, from https://www.unhcr.org/news/latest/2017/9/59ba9b7b4/rohingya-influx-strains-camp-resources-bangladesh.html

UNHCR Bangladesh. (n.d.). *Operational response dashboard on Myanmar Refugees*. Author. Retrieved May 5, 2021, from https://data2.unhcr.org/en/documents/details/60981

UNICEF. (2019). *Multiple indicator cluster survey 2019*. UNICEF and Bangladesh Bureau of Statistics. Retrieved from www.unicef.org/bangladesh/media/3281/file/Bangladesh%202019%20MICS%20Report_English.pdf

UNICEF. (n.d.). *Core commitments to children*. Author. Retrieved January 1, 2021, from https://www.unicef.org/emergencies/core-commitments-children

UNICEF and IPA. (2018). *Baseline survey to assess/monitor current level of knowledge, attitudes, practices, and behaviors (KAPB) of the Rohingyas and Host Community in Cox's Bazar, study report*. UNICEF. Retrieved from https://www.unicef.org/bangladesh/en/reports/knowledge-attitudes-practices-and-behaviours-rohingya-and-host-communities-coxs-bazar

UNICEF and IPA. (2019). *Midline survey to assess/monitor current level of knowledge, attitudes, practices, and behaviors (KAPB) of the Rohingyas and Host Community in Cox's Bazar*. UNICEF. Unpublished.

Vandenent, M., Minjoon K., Johnstone, D., Kapil, N., Metenier, J., Widiati, Y., Hasan, M., Worth, M., Bhatnagar, A., Khan A. I., Qadri, F., & Khan, A., Faruque (2019) Public health challenges to combat cholera in humanitarian crisis: Experiences from Rohingya crisis. Presented at 15th Asian Conference on Diarrhoeal Disease and Nutrition (ASCODD 2020), 28–30th January.

WHO. (2018). *Bangladesh: Rohingya Refugee crisis 2017–2018. Public health situation analysis*. Author. Retrieved from https://www.who.int/docs/default-source/searo/bangladesh/bangladesh%2D%2D-rohingya-crisis%2D%2D-pdf-reports/public-health-situation-analysis-may-2018.pdf?Status=Temp&sfvrsn=9a280761_2

World Bank. (2016). *Bangladesh interactive poverty map*. Author. Retrieved December 19, 2020, from https://www.worldbank.org/en/data/interactive/2016/11/10/bangladesh-poverty-maps

World Humanitarian Summit. (n.d.). Retrieved December 19, 2020, from https://agendaforhumanity.org/summit.html

Part III
Lessons Learned: Conclusions and Recommendations

Chapter 10
Reflections and Recommendations for Future Disease Outbreak and Pandemic Response

Ketan Chitnis, Rafael Obregon, and Erma Manoncourt

Contents

Introduction

The collection of chapters featured in this book provide important insights about the increasing complexity of preparedness and response to infectious disease outbreaks and pandemics, with a particular emphasis on the role of communication and community engagement and on the need to broaden our understanding of how a wide range of social, political, cultural, rights and communication dynamics and issues should inform communication and community engagement in current and future responses. Further, these insights have relevant conceptual, policy and programmatic implications for public health decision makers and practitioners and for the global public health community as a whole. In this chapter, we draw on this collection of chapters and put forward: (a) our own reflections about the current status of addressing complex human behaviour in responding to disease outbreaks,

K. Chitnis (✉)
UNICEF Mozambique, Maputo, Mozambique

R. Obregon
UNICEF, Asunción, Paraguay

E. Manoncourt
Management & Development Consulting, Inc., Las Vegas, NV, USA

E. Manoncourt et al. (eds.), *Communication and Community Engagement in Disease Outbreaks*, https://doi.org/10.1007/978-3-030-92296-2_10

epidemics and pandemics, and (b) recommendations for ongoing and future responses, which cut across conceptual, policy and programmatic issues.

Reflections

Risk Communication and Community Engagement

While global- and country-level discussions in wealthier countries point to unprecedented investments to develop vaccines that may help preempt other outbreaks with global implications and the potential to threaten humanity, the unpredictable nature of viruses such as the COVID-19 means that serious investments are also needed to strengthen risk communication and community engagement efforts as a key strategy. COVID-19 and Ebola, and previous outbreaks, have shown that even the availability of vaccines does not guarantee their widespread availability and acceptability and that engagement of communities and public trust will remain central to any immunization effort.

We note that there has been an increasing recognition of, and investments made to use rapid socio-anthropological research to improve the efficacy of risk communication and community engagement in recent years. The focus of this rapid evidence generation has been to unpack a range of complex social factors that determine human behaviour, be it individual or collective behaviours, as well as to understand government response to outbreaks (Carter et al., 2021). The topics covered have been exhaustive, from migration patterns to gender norms to local understanding of disease transmission and prevention. Such insights have informed and improved public health responses. Yet an area that continues to face challenges is evidence generation that is led by local communities. Experiences of locally owned and led social science research processes to promote contextualized solutions for prevention, containment and ending of an outbreak are not widespread. Investments in local socio-anthropological and communication research capacity and establishment of local networks and south-south collaboration teams similar to global collaboration but adapted to regional, sub-regional and country-specific contexts with optimal financing should be prioritized.

Another area where there is consensus at a normative level but where major gaps remain is the systematic understanding and implementation of community engagement. Operationalizing community engagement as a locally led, community-driven and decentralized process, and a strategy needs rethinking at all levels. While there is a great deal of talk and discussion about the importance of community engagement, it is not necessarily put in practice at the scale that is needed (Rohan & McKay, 2021). There are multiple reasons for this. They include, among others, governments often dictating response strategies in the larger public interest, the need to demonstrate swift action or to respond to external funding demands with conditionalities and short timeframes to contain an outbreak, and the lack of local level commitment and leadership to devise community-owned solutions. While minimum standards for community engagement have recently been developed as explained by Bedson and Abramowitz in Chap. 3 in this book, its uptake among donors, agencies, governments and awareness about such standards among local communities themselves is yet to take place. There is a need for an even stronger push to require public health strategies to bring communities to the forefront of outbreak response and to mainstream this practice into health systems. After all, 'the public' in public health is about people and communities, and in order to have trust, confidence, respect for human rights and to counter mis- and dis-information, community engagement is perhaps the only vaccine.

Several case studies included in this book provide examples of locally initiated actions at community level to curb the spread of infectious diseases; however, these initiatives are not always at the core of national response strategies. More efforts are needed to demonstrate evidence of community-owned and locally contextualized interventions and processes replicated at scale in a given context. Such kind of evidence is not only critical to public health response but also to demonstrate how it contributes to building trust, how community resilience is critical to curbing transmission and to show the key role of social cohesion to deal with uncertainty and to make sense of the evolving science about outbreaks.

Culture

We note the tension between balancing bio-medical advice on preventive behaviours for short or medium term to help contain the spread of an infectious disease with the prevailing cultural practices and social context. Understanding, adapting, recasting and negotiating preventive behaviours remain challenging for outbreak response teams and large segments of the population in any society. This is especially the case with the most vulnerable and hard-to-reach groups due to the need for translating concepts and actions needed into local and native languages, especially those with limited resources and those without a written form. Added to this, low levels of literacy, poor access to communication platforms, especially digital, and the difficulties inherent to promoting behaviour change, often in short periods of time, need deeper understanding of and negotiation with local communities about strongly rooted cultural practices.

Another relevant aspect of culture illustrated by some of the case studies is the current lack of gender sensitive responses to outbreak response. While the singular focus on interrupting disease transmission makes sense from an epidemiological perspective, often the burden of protective household behaviours adds more work to women, including girls, who are already overworked being primary caregivers. This was noted in the experience of Zika control in Latin America, among the refugee Rohingya women in Bangladesh, in Ebola control in West Africa and more recently in the COVID-19 response across many countries and regions (Power, 2020).

While the focus of social science-based interventions is to communicate the risk and to promote appropriate preventive behaviours at community level, they also need to pay attention to limiting transmission from those infected at home to other family members, an issue that became critical in the Ebola outbreaks and the COVID-19 pandemic. In this context, disease outbreak strategies need to factor in more explicitly socio-cultural aspects for the provision of care at home or in healthcare settings by family members. Strategies also need to have a deeper understanding of funerary and/or burial practices by considering rituals related to handling deceased family members, which often become drivers for disease transmission. While Ebola in West Africa brought these aspects into sharp relief, we believe, however, that more social science and behavioural science informed practice is needed to address these issues in future disease outbreak responses.

Complexity

Controlling an outbreak while minimizing its socio-economic impact on affected communities requires further social and behavioural investigation and a more nuanced guidance to addressing those factors. Short-term behaviour change to limit the spread of a disease, for instance, makes imminent sense from a public health angle, but the close link between diseases and livelihoods needs to be factored in more substantively in designing prevention and response strategies. This has been recognized by officials, yet we believe that such intersections between people, diseases, livelihoods and economy are not sufficiently informing disease control strategies.

While the current COVID-19 pandemic is an extreme event in terms of its impact on the global and local economy, given the increasing threat posed by climate change, the ongoing globalization with increased trade and travel and the growing animal to human interaction due to changing demographics and urbanization, experts are raising the concern of more frequent epidemics and pandemics (The Lancet Microbe, 2021). Given these trends, disease, epidemics and pandemic preparedness, and response strategies need to factor in complex factors that impact all facets of individual and societal life, and avoid the use only of an individual or collective behaviour change and risk communication lens to public health response.

Beyond the socio-economic impact during disease outbreaks, complexity also needs to tackle pre-outbreak social factors such as investment in systems and platforms as preparedness measures that can be quickly mobilized during outbreaks—small or large. Here, social science interventions for public health like the ones presented in this book need greater attention and investments as part of systems strengthening efforts in all countries. Much like efforts to strengthening surveillance, laboratory capacities and health workforce to detect, identify and track outbreaks, complexity in public health should take a 'whole of society' approach.

Human Rights

Pandemics and outbreaks such as COVID-19 and Ebola have brought to the forefront the challenges that the intersection of human rights and outbreak response increasingly pose to governments, civil society and communities. Some of the restrictions introduced to contain and control these outbreaks and pandemics, which have been considered necessary from a public health perspective, such as quarantines, lockdowns and curfews, closing of borders, suspension of flights, definitions about essential activities that prevented many from working, are seen by many as violations of their individual rights.

Human rights violations have been reported and discussed across many countries during the COVID-19 (Lebret, 2020; Spadaro, 2020) especially for groups such as migrant workers (when sudden local and international borders were closed), children (due to long-term school closures and billions without reliable access to remote learning) and adolescents, especially adolescent girls (school dropout, exposure to violence at home and child marriage) and people living with disabilities (sign language when using masks), among other groups.

While disease outbreaks supersede human rights in the interest of larger public good, how do we balance individual and collective rights and address rights violations in the future? This area of work needs rethinking and agenda setting at its highest level in terms of global health security, strong and expanded social protection programmes, normative guidelines that govern international and national responses, and the application of international law for movement of people and goods.

Trust

While community engagement is widely talked about in the context of disease outbreaks and pandemics, in the end it is the public and individual trust across different levels that truly makes or breaks the effectiveness of preparedness and response (Larson & Heymann, 2010; Ryan, et al., 2019). Trust is very hard to build but very easy to lose, especially in emergency and crisis situations, and in situations where there has not been enough effort invested between the government authorities, the public health responders and the different communities.

Transparent, timely and effective two-way communication is one part of building trust; however, there are other facets to it as well such as active listening; respect of local knowledge, culture and decision-making; and being adaptive to changing circumstances and evolving science. In essence, building and maintaining trust is a dynamic process that needs to be closely monitored and addressed.

We note that effective health outbreak strategies do pay attention to building trust; however, they rely mostly on providing accurate information through technical teams and through risk communication experts to avoid and manage crises. We believe that building trust in disease outbreak response is everyone's responsibility, especially all those involved in engaging directly with communities (Enria, et al., 2021). Investments in capacity building and training are, therefore, needed for all responders engaged in efforts to implement culturally appropriate and responsive communication.

Infodemics

With a plethora of real-time, user generated and widely disseminated communication platforms available, information about new disease outbreaks is plentiful. However, this also often leads to an information overload, and it makes it hard for people to distinguish factually correct information and public health advice from misinformation and rumors that are circulated due to lack of understanding of the facts or to some other extraneous factors. To add to this, there are also small groups of people that are vested in promoting disinformation about disease outbreaks, as well as its origins and how to protect oneself. This disinformation is also circulating on perhaps the same communication platforms which are used by public health responders.

As public health professionals we want to promote transparency, build trust, be culturally relevant and sensitive and communicate fact-based information about disease transmission and how to protect oneself, but there will likely be conspiracy theories and a proliferation of factually incorrect information that should be addressed head-on through the engagement of communities that may believe in such misinformation. Plus, the channels and platforms that promote disinformation need to be acknowledged and addressed. Machine learning, artificial intelligence and bots could be used in real time and at scale to pull down misinformation and disinformation circulating on social media and websites (Tsao, et al., 2021). This will require large-scale efforts to enforce stricter information communication laws internationally and to ensure optimal investments to identify and tackle such sources on a routine basis.

We believe that cultivating relationships through extensive community engagement and building support for well-respected and credible information channels needs proactive approaches. Building those relationships during a public health emergency is a challenging task. On the one hand, sustained partnerships with credible sources such as news and pro-social entertainment media are needed. On the other hand, proactive ways to track social media through tools such as social listening also need to be widely used for decision-making. As members of a global community of scholars and practitioners, we need to develop newer approaches and strategies to deal with misinformation and disinformation as part of a routine practice of improving communication and community engagement intervention for disease outbreak, epidemic and pandemic response.

Recommendations

Based on lessons learned from the case studies discussed in the preceding chapters and building upon the aforementioned reflections, the following recommendations are made to inform academics, researchers, practitioners and decision-makers as part of ongoing and future praxis on disease outbreak communication and broader outbreak, epidemic and pandemic preparedness and response strategies.

Policy Decisions and Implementation

Despite some progress in the past few years, preparedness for disease outbreaks and pandemics is largely under-valued and under-funded, especially when it comes to the role of social science and communication and community engagement considerations in public health. For communication and community engagement strategies for future disease outbreaks to be better managed, greater considerations need to be given to topics such as building and maintaining trust, balancing scientifically sound information with cultural nuances and community concerns, and delivering timely information while being nimble in providing new evidence and facts and in managing infodemics. We call upon decision-makers to pay attention to this gap.

The discourse and action on global health security and pandemic preparedness should give even more prominence to social science and communication and community engagement as part of a comprehensive socio-bio-medical approach. Medical innovations, faster data sharing, surveillance, laboratory capacities, therapeutic and vaccines are critical to being better prepared for future outbreaks and pandemics. However, trying to do damage control after the disease outbreak crisis unfolds is too costly as lives and economies are at stake often due to the lack of correct and culturally relevant information on prevention, confusion as a result of infodemics and deep distrust in authorities managing outbreaks. Hence, we urge the global health community and public health policy-makers to pay greater attention to socio-cultural and complexity-driven solutions. This will only be possible through the enactment of comprehensive national policies and initiatives aimed at strengthening capacities on social science and communication and engagement in public health at national and, especially, local levels that are adequately funded and resourced.

Social Science Research in Pandemics and Disease Outbreaks

Research in key social and behavioural areas of pandemic preparedness and response such as gender and culture require greater attention, especially at national and local levels. Gender aspects, while critically important in responding to most outbreaks covered in this book, namely Zika, COVID-19 and Ebola, among others, continue to be under-researched to inform social science and communication and engagement interventions and are often absent in programmatic considerations and implementation. The role of women in preventive practices, as care providers to children and other family members and in shaping community resilience and response, needs more recognition and support from public health policies, researchers and practitioners. Furthermore, how pandemics impact women and girls need to be better understood and the implementation of gender-sensitive interventions needs to be strengthened. The challenges of integrating gender more effectively in preparedness and response are also applicable to other factors that often generate greater vulnerability to pandemics, especially issues such as disability, ethnicity and language. Researchers should increasingly fill these gaps with social science evidence.

Cultural nuances and the role of local languages that influence understanding, control and prevention of disease transmission are also lacking robust evidence. Preventive strategies will not be successful or will lead to resistance from communities unless they are contextualized and, ideally, co-designed with communities. Failures as a result of top-down interventions are well documented, but more evidence is needed to demonstrate how investments in research on socio-cultural aspects that foreground communities in the response strategies can be done at scale to benefit public health approaches. This type of work requires substantive investments, especially at the local level.

Investments are also needed to enhance national capacity to conduct and rapidly use social science research, especially in countries that face recurring disease outbreaks. We call upon donors, practitioners and researchers who have supported, managed or conducted this type of research to continue nurturing local or regional networks, which can be leveraged for future outbreaks or to inform preparedness measures. It is worth mentioning, however, that better use of social science research is often related not only to the availability of national technical capacities but also to the availability of resources to build and strengthen a reliable human resource capacity base that can consistently generate quality and reliable data and evidence. Long-term partnerships that connect global, national and local capacities is critical to move forward in this area. We therefore urge more attention to social science research capacity building, partnerships and global to local networking to generate and use data to inform disease outbreaks management and control.

Practice Related to Risk Communication and Community Engagement for Pandemics and Disease Outbreaks

While the function and role of communication and community engagement is well-recognized and is increasingly mainstreamed in global and national guidance to manage disease outbreaks, systems and capacities to design and manage large-scale interventions alongside biomedical strategies, still remain weak or incipient in many countries. We urge a systems strengthening approach to communication and community engagement that goes down to local administrative level in terms of planning and implementing strategies. Some good examples that can inform future practice come from programmes such as social mobilization and behaviour change for polio eradication and the implementation of communication strategies for HIV/AIDS prevention and care seeking. These well-documented examples prioritized all or a combination of communication and community engagement strategies that should serve as a model for current and future public health threats. Practitioners should look back, learn from the past and design communication and engagement approaches needed today. While the field of practice continues to evolve with new ways of communication and changing community dynamics, core principles to embed the function of communication and engagement within institutional structures remains. Further, several considerations included in Chap. 2, about the global architecture of risk communication and community engagement, provide practical entry points to address what we believe is the fundamental challenge—localized capacity. We urge policy-makers and practitioners to address this gap.

Donor Prioritization for Community-Driven Preparedness, Control and Response

Investments in the broader field of social science, including areas covered in this book such as risk communication, community engagement, culture, trust, human rights, complexity and infodemics, are increasing but are not at the level that is needed. We urge donors to do more on their part by requiring funding proposals and initiatives funded through direct support to governments and agencies to explicitly outline how the social science in disease outbreak practice will be prioritized.

This call comes from the lessons we have documented in the case studies in this book and from other reports from Ebola prevention to COVID-19 that highlight why public health responders need to build trust with communities, address risk perceptions including misinformation and dis-information, promote community ownership and address gendered roles and cultural nuances among others for programmes to be successful. While a call for additional investments may not sound appealing, the reality is that the cost of strengthening national, and especially local capacities, to address pandemics and large-scale outbreaks in the long run is arguably a fraction of the cost of responding to outbreaks, as demonstrated by past experience from avian influenza to most recently from COVID-19. We urge donors to pay attention to this area.

Coordination Between Governments, Implementing Agencies and Community Networks

While improved coordination has been documented between governments and agencies supporting public health responders at international, national and sub-national levels, there is a need to rethink the role of communities in this work. We believe that for complex and long-lasting outbreaks and pandemics, coordination structures have largely failed to be sustained after the initial phase of the response. This leads to duplication of efforts, wastage of precious resources and lack of attention to needs of communities. We therefore call upon government authorities to consider coordination of social science informed interventions to be institutionalized within national bodies, under the leadership of a clearly appointed lead agency or institution. In addition, coordination works best at the local level given that social science researchers, communication and engagement practitioners, and other public health responders are closest to the communities. Therefore, we urge governments to ensure that community networks play an active role within local coordination structures to improve accountability to those most impacted by outbreaks.

Conclusion

The collection of chapters in this book includes a rich mix of conceptual and practice-based contributions that collectively provide critical insights towards strengthening the role of communication and engagement to address social and behavioural determinants in pandemic and disease outbreak preparedness and response. We believe that the proposal to consider an integrated conceptual framework that makes justice to the complexity of social and behavioural dimensions of pandemic and disease outbreak preparedness and response is broadly supported by the accounts, findings and recommendations of the wide range of contributions and experiences included in the book. The extent to which this can be taken one step further will depend upon initiatives that field test the expanded framework or that at least apply it through specific interventions.

We recognize, however, that several challenges remain. First, the natural tendency to seek technological solutions anchored in vaccines, diagnostics and treatments is very powerful in global efforts to address any disease outbreak. The reasons for this are well known. However, the case studies featured in this book across a number of infectious disease outbreaks individually and collectively reveal, to a large extent, that social and behavioural aspects of pandemic preparedness and response and non-pharmaceutical interventions are already at the heart of it and that in some cases, they have been the first line of defence. Second, the tendency to 'prioritize and forget' seems to be a recurrent practice. Once outbreaks get out of control or that standard biomedical responses are not sufficient, calls for greater investments and focus on communication and community engagement emerge, only for it to quickly take a back seat once the outbreak has been brought under relative control. Third, the persistent gap between the global and the national and local, wherein global frameworks, technical guidance and protocols, and technical support, among other tools, are not consistently applied at local levels. Communication and community engagement need to find its place in the architecture of global and national health systems in terms that are equal to other components of it.

As long as communication and community engagement remain critical to the prevention, control and response of pandemics and disease outbreaks, we will be compelled to continue advocating for greater investments and attention from policymakers, researchers, practitioners and donors to ensure that the public and communities are fully engaged and are at the centre of pandemic and disease outbreak preparedness and response. We truly hope that this book contributes to that effort.

Disclaimer The views expressed in this chapter are those of the authors and do not represent the official position of UNICEF.

References

Carter, S. E., Ahuka-Mundeke, S., Pfaffmann Zambruni, J., et al. (2021). How to improve outbreak response: A case study of integrated outbreak analytics from Ebola in Eastern Democratic Republic of the Congo. *BMJ Global Health, 6*, e006736.

Enria, L., Waterlow, N., Rogers, N. T., Brindle, H., Lal, S., Eggo, R. M., Lees, S., & Roberts, C. H. (2021). Trust and transparency in times of crisis: Results from an online survey during the first wave (April 2020) of the COVID-19 epidemic in the UK. *PLOS ONE, 16*(2), e0239247. https://doi.org/10.1371/journal.pone.0239247

Larson, H. J. (2010). Public Health Response to Influenza A(H1N1) as an Opportunity to Build Public Trust. *JAMA, 303*(3), 271. https://doi.org/10.1001/jama.2009.2023

Lebret, A. (2020). COVID-19 pandemic and derogation to human rights. *Journal of Law and the Biosciences, 7*(1), lsaa015. https://doi.org/10.1093/jlb/lsaa015

Power, K. (2020). The COVID-19 pandemic has increased the care burden of women and families. *Sustainability: Science, Practice and Policy, 16*(1), 67–73. https://doi.org/10.1080/15487733.2020.1776561

Ryan, M. J., Giles-Vernick, T., & Graham, J. E. (2019). Technologies of trust in epidemic response: openness, reflexivity and accountability during the 2014–2016 Ebola outbreak in West Africa. *BMJ Global Health, 4*(1), e001272. https://doi.org/10.1136/bmjgh-2018-001272

Rohan, H., & McKay, G. (2021). The Ebola outbreak in the Democratic Republic of the Congo: Why there is no 'silver bullet'. *Nature Immunology, 21*, 591–594. https://doi.org/10.1038/s41590-020-0675-8

Spadaro, A. (2020). COVID-19: Testing the limits of human rights. *European Journal of Risk Regulation, 11*(2), 317–325. https://doi.org/10.1017/err.2020.27

The Lancet Microbe. (2021). Climate change: fires, floods, and infectious diseases. The Lancet Microbe, 2(9), e415. https://doi.org/10.1016/s2666-5247(21)00220-2

Tsao, S. F., Chen, H., Tisseverasinghe, T., Yang, Y., Li, L., & Butt, Z. A. (2021). What social media told us in the time of COVID-19: a scoping review. *The Lancet Digital Health, 3*(3), e175–e194. https://doi.org/10.1016/s2589-7500(20)30315-0

Index

E. Manoncourt et al. (eds.), *Communication and Community Engagement in Disease Outbreaks*, https://doi.org/10.1007/978-3-030-92296-2

The manufacturer's authorised representative in the EU is Springer Nature Customer Service Centre GmbH, Europaplatz 3, 69115 Heidelberg, Germany. If you have any concerns regarding our products, please contact ProductSafety@springernature.com

Printed and bound by CPI Group (UK) Ltd, Croydon, CR0 4YY

30/09/2026

02225291-0003